£2

PRACTICAL DERMATOLOGY

PRACTICAL DERMATOLOGY

BY

I. B. SNEDDON
M.B., Ch.B., F.R.C.P.

*Consultant Dermatologist, Rupert Hallam Department of
Dermatology United Sheffield Hospitals;
Hon. Clinical Lecturer in Dermatology
University of Sheffield*

and

R. E. CHURCH
M.A., M.D., B.Ch., F.R.C.P.Ed.

*Consultant Dermatologist, Rupert Hallam Department of
Dermatology, United Sheffield Hospitals;
Hon. Clinical Lecturer in Dermatology
University of Sheffield*

EDWARD ARNOLD

© I. B. Sneddon and R. E. Church 1971

First published 1964
by Edward Arnold (Publishers) Ltd
25 Hill Street,
London, W1X 8LL

Reprinted 1966
Reprinted 1968
Reprinted 1970

Second Edition 1971
Reprinted 1972

ISBN: 0 7131 4183 2

Set in 10 on 11 pt. Monotype Plantin, printed by letterpress,
and bound in Great Britain at The Pitman Press, Bath

PREFACE TO SECOND EDITION

WE have been encouraged by the reception of the first edition to undertake the task of revision. We are most grateful for the criticisms and helpful suggestions made by our colleagues at home and overseas, many of which have been acted upon.

Much research in Dermatology in the last five years has advanced the knowledge of the biology of the skin and the pathology of its disorders. We have been relieved to find few major changes in the practical management of the common skin complaints. Perhaps an awareness of the many undesirable effects of treatment has been the greatest advance.

Our decision to limit advice on treatment to those methods with which we are familiar has been maintained and the temptation to enlarge the book beyond its orginal scope has been resisted.

We are especially grateful to the Chief Pharmacist of the Hallamshire Hospital, Mr. J. D. Cronin, for his patience and constant advice on pharmaceutical problems, and we are also, as always, indebted to our secretaries.

I.B.S.
R.E.C.

Sheffield, 1971

v

PREFACE TO FIRST EDITION

THIS book is an adaptation of lectures given to Undergraduate students and General Practitioner Refresher courses in the University of Sheffield.

The space allotted to any subject has been based mainly on its incidence in general practice and in the out patient department. A few rare diseases have been included either because harm would befall the patient if their diagnosis was missed or because they illustrate vividly a biological principle.

Clinical descriptions have been curtailed because it is our belief that practical experience is the only way in which the differential diagnosis of skin diseases can be learnt, and it is hoped that the book will be used as an adjunct to clinical teaching.

The advice on treatment is dogmatic but based only on treatment which we have ourselves tried and found to be satisfactory.

We are indebted to Mr. A. S. Foster, Medical Artist, Mr. G. Swann of the Department of Photography, Royal Infirmary, Sheffield, and our secretaries, Mrs. B. V. Coombe, Miss Rita Carr and Mrs. B. Bell, without whose assistance the book would never have been completed. Lastly and by no means least we are grateful to our wives for suffering many evenings in silence.

CONTENTS

CHAPTER I

THE APPROACH TO THE SKIN PATIENT

THE doctor who treats diseases of the skin is at a disadvantage compared with his colleagues in other branches of medicine. He deals with an organ which can be seen and felt, and it is impossible to hoodwink a patient into thinking that the complaint has improved when obviously it has not. Many patients with skin disease believe that because the lesion is on the surface it should be easy to cure and any failure in treatment implies that his doctor is a fool. The patient who has spent a sleepless night because of an irritation is highly critical and even aggressive towards his doctor, and it is this feeling of blameworthiness in the doctor which increases his difficulties.

There is a great temptation to change treatment needlessly and start the great evil of dermatology, over-treatment. Few doctors, other than trained specialists, have confidence in their ability to diagnose and treat skin conditions and this lack of confidence is soon conveyed to the patient. Yet the diagnosis and management of the common skin disorders is not particularly difficult and allows the doctor to play detective more than many other branches of medicine.

The skin is part of the whole being and changes in it may reflect systemic or psychological disorders. Accurate observation of the skin may, therefore, assist in the diagnosis of general disease.

History

The foundation stone of the diagnosis is the history. Not only can the correct diagnosis be frequently deduced from the history alone, but some assessment of the personality of the patient can be made. It is permissible to have a brief glance at the lesion of which the patient complains in order to save time. Obviously, if the patient has a wart on the hand or a rodent ulcer on the face, there is no point in taking a lengthy history, but for most skin eruptions, a comprehensive history before a full examination is advisable. The duration of disease, the first site affected and the mode of subsequent spread should be elicited. What has been applied by the patient? The majority try several remedies before consulting a doctor and are unwilling to admit this, yet the whole character of a skin eruption can be masked by a reaction to local applications. Are there symptoms from the rash? Does it itch or burn and if so, is it worse at any particular time? The itching of scabies is particularly noticeable at night whereas chronic urticaria is most severe on waking. Is there a previous history of skin disease?

The same type as the present, or was it different? Are other members of the family affected? A positive answer suggests either contagious disease or a genetic disorder. Have other members of the family suffered from hay fever, asthma or urticaria? These diseases are known to be associated with chronic eczema. What is the patient's occupation? It is not sufficient to discover that he is a turner, many skin conditions arise from contact with substances which slowly damage the skin and it is important to know exactly what has happened at work; as in the case of a turner, what metals are being turned? Is the lathe lubricated with soluble oil? How are the hands protected and cleaned? Has the patient hobbies which entail contact with skin irritants? If a man, does he help with the washing up or home decorating? What is the patient's general health, has he been able to sleep, or has he been mentally irritable or depressed? Are medicines of any type being taken? Here it may be necessary to ask leading questions since patients do not remember aspirins, routine sleeping tablets and aperients. Finally, it is always worth while asking the patient for his or her theories for the cause of the complaint. Often these are erroneous, sometimes humorous, but a useful clue may be provided. It also gives a guide to the patient's knowledge of medicine which will be helpful in later discussion of the complaint.

Having taken the history, a diagnosis may be suggested, certainly some will be excluded. For instance, if the eruption has been present ten years a self-limiting virus infection, lasting a few weeks, is an impossibility.

The examination

Except where the diagnosis is obvious and trivial, such as a simple wart, the patient must be undressed and examined completely, preferably in daylight since small degrees of colour variation are not easily seen in artificial light. Complete examination should be insisted on since it is a frequent occurrence for a patient to deny that there are any lesions on the covered parts of the body and yet on complete examination an eruption is found. This is not always a result of deliberate deception. A mild dermatitis of the eyelids is often the first sign of a generalised allergic reaction to nickel suspenders, yet a woman patient will not mention that she has a rash on the thighs because she does not associate the rash on the thighs with that on the eyelids. A complete examination will reveal the eruption and provide the clue for the correct diagnosis. Another common association is between the hands and feet. Fungus infection of the toes often causes an eruption on the hands, therefore no examination of a rash on the hands is satisfactory unless the feet are also examined. The scalp, the nails and the mucous membranes are all part of the skin and must be included in the examination. Any enlargement of superficial lymphatic glands should be noted. Always remember it is the whole patient that is being examined and take note of abnormalities in other organs than the skin.

The skin lesions

In order to discuss changes in the skin, it is necessary to have a standard descriptive terminology and when examining a rash an attempt should be made to find the earliest lesion and to define this. A *macule* is a localised change in colour of the skin with no elevation or infiltration, a common example is a freckle, but macules can be erythematous,

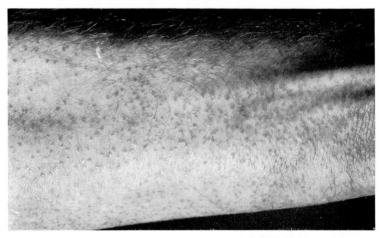

Fig. 1.—Distinct papules in a case of lichen nitidus.

purpuric or pigmented. A *papule* is a small solid elevation; papules can be flat topped or conical, round or polyhedral, follicular when related to hair follicles, smooth or scaly. A *vesicle* is a small collection of fluid either in the epidermis or between the epidermis and dermis. It may be difficult to determine whether an elevated lesion is a papule or a vesicle and in eczematous eruptions there is a transition from papule to vesicle. A *pustule* is a superficial collection of pus in the skin and pustules may form as a result of purulent change in a vesicle or *de novo*. A *bulla* is a collection of fluid larger than a vesicle the roof of which may be the whole or part of the epidermis. A *wheal* is a transient elevation of the skin caused by oedema in the dermis and surrounding capillary dilatation.

Certain secondary changes may result from the primary lesions. *Scales* which are heaped up horny layer or dead epidermis may develop as a result of inflammatory changes. If serum, pus or blood dry on the

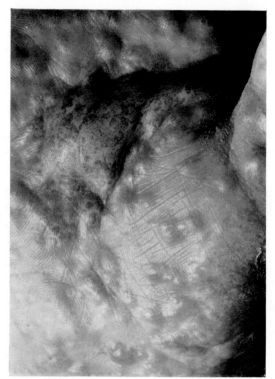

FIG. 2.—Vesicles in contact dermatitis of hand. The vesicles in the centre have formed a multilocular bulla.

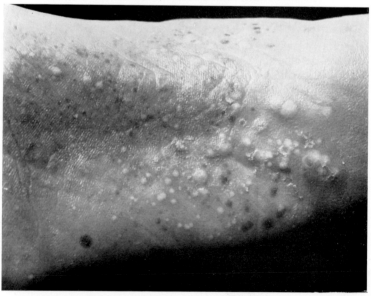

FIG. 3.—Pustules on the sole in psoriasis.

skin *crusts* are formed. *Fissures* and *cracks* occur in skin folds and where inflamed thickened inelastic skin moves over joints. Superficial loss of skin or mucous membranes gives rise to *erosions*, deeper loss is described as *ulceration*. An aggregation of chronic inflammatory cells in the dermis, such as occurs in chronic infection with tuberculosis or leprosy,

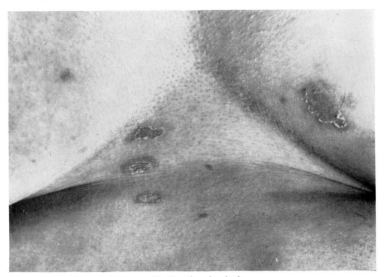

FIG. 4.—Scaling in pityriasis rosea.

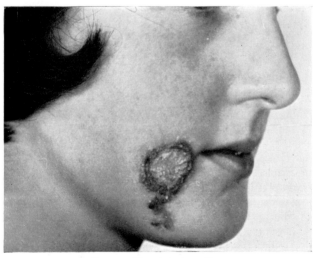

FIG. 5.—Crusts in impetigo.

gives rise to a translucent papule usually of yellowish-brown hue. Such change is termed a granulomatous reaction and a very similar appearance is given by infiltration with neoplastic cells.

Having identified the type of lesion affecting the skin, much can be learned from its distribution. This can best be assessed from a distance of 6 feet. On the whole, endogenous eruptions are symmetrical,

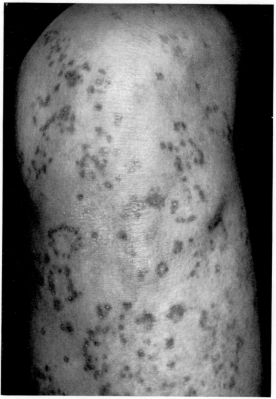

FIG. 6.—Translucent papules of a granuloma (sarcoidosis).

affecting mirror image areas. Psoriasis affects the extensor aspects of the limbs whilst lichen planus more often involves the flexor surfaces. It may be that only those parts of the skin exposed to light are inflamed, in that case, the back of the hands, the face, the V of the neck, but not the area beneath the chin, will be affected. A few congenital abnormalities have a segmental distribution but the common unilateral segmental eruption is herpes zoster which appears on the skin supplied by one cutaneous nerve root. Purely linear lesions suggest plant sensitivity, artefact or the Koebner phenomenon, in which skin damage by a scratch may be the site of an endogenous eruption such as psoriasis or lichen planus. Certain diseases have unique features such as the burrow of scabies or the umbilicated nodule of molluscum contagiosum and when they are found the diagnosis is not in doubt.

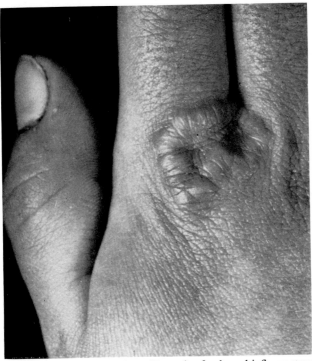

Fig. 7.—Granuloma annulare. Example of a dermal inflammatory collagen disorder.

Even with the most careful history and examination, a definite diagnosis may not be possible. There are many investigative procedures which can then assist and of these, histological examination of a piece of skin (biopsy) is the most important. Bacteriological and mycological examination of pus, scales or hair and investigation of the patients' blood or urine, may all be necessary. If allergic contact dermatitis is suspected patch tests will be required to confirm specific sensitivity.

Finally, observation over a period of time may provide the solution. The diagnosis of a lesion which on first appearance is atypical or misleading may, in its later stages, appear obvious. Patients with contact dermatitis often cannot, at the first interview, remember all the substances they have handled; at a subsequent interview the cause may be recalled with ease.

Having attained a diagnosis, the disease must be viewed against the background of the individual. There may be no problem if a patient has only a simple infection easily controlled by topical treatment but there are many factors to consider in, for instance, a housewife's dermatitis. In this condition the skin of the hands becomes red, cracked and irritable owing to excessive contact with soap or detergents and water. There may be an hereditary weakness which will be shown by a history of skin disease in relatives. Previous attacks or an undue dryness of the skin of the rest of the body denote a constitutional liability. A recent difference in the degree of contact with soap and water may have occurred; perhaps the patient has just had a baby or has been widowed and has had to do extra domestic work. The skin is more likely to break down if poorly nourished and thus anaemia or malnutrition may be factors. Skin damage appears more often during hormonal changes such as the menopause and in old age. It is probable that the general state of tissue irritability and the sweating mechanisms can also be altered by emotional tension. Emotional upsets certainly influence symptoms and the complaint will thus be aggravated by unhappiness, anxiety and depression. It can be seen, therefore, that what seems a relatively simple problem is the end result of many contributory factors. Housewives' dermatitis has been taken as an example but similar factors are at work in many patients with skin disease. Many will recover with use of routine treatment but in order to achieve the best result an attempt should be made to correct as many other contributory factors as possible.

As mentioned before, the big danger in the management of skin diseases is over-treatment. This term means irritation of the skin by applications which in themselves are irritants, applied too frequently and cleaned off too vigorously. From the treatment aspect skin eruptions can be classified into four main groups—

(1) Those which if protected from the doctor and the patient will recover.
(2) Those conditions which require skin rest by the application of inert and soothing preparations.
(3) Infections which need a specific antibiotic or fungicide.
(4) Those diseases which in the present state of our knowledge are uninfluenced by treatment.

When in doubt use the simplest and safest applications is the maxim to be kept constantly in mind.

Patients with skin disease are more disturbed by their complaint than patients with other medical disorders. Skin eruptions still produce the leper complex, a feeling of shame, disgust and fear and it is this emotional state which adds to the difficulty of the management of skin patients. Irritation, which is such a constant symptom of skin disease, disturbs sleep and is frequently more lowering to the morale than pain. Fear that the disease is contagious and will spread to relatives and friends adds to the patient's misery.

If these fears are recognised by the doctor and discussed, even though they are not voiced by the patient, anxiety will be lessened and this can only be beneficial whatever the dermatosis. Fear is the motive which brings many patients for consultation and even though the skin complaint may be incurable the fact that the disease is recognised and its natural history is known relieves symptoms in a surprisingly high proportion of patients.

CHAPTER 2

THE STRUCTURE OF THE SKIN

THE skin consists of two layers, the epidermis derived from the embryo-logical ectoderm and the dermis or corium which is of mesodermal origin. The epidermis is a many layered pavement of squamous epithelial cells devoid of blood vessels and nourished by a plexus of capillaries situated in the upper or papillary part of the dermis. Although the epidermis can be divided morphologically into four different layers—the horny, granular, prickle cell and, the lowest, the basal layer—each level in the skin represents a stage in the life of the epidermal cell.

The columnar cells of the basal or germinal layer give rise to the prickle cells by cell division. These polygonal cells are intimately connected to their neighbours by protoplasmic fibrils or prickles. The

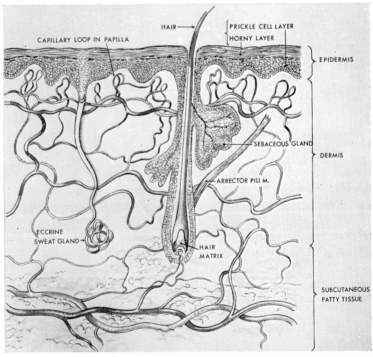

FIG. 8.—Diagram of the main structures of the skin.

prickle cells move upwards to the surface as new cells are formed beneath them. As they approach the surface they take on their primary function of producing the protective material, keratin. It is the physico-chemical changes taking place in the cells preparatory to keratinisation which produce the granular layer. Finally, the epidermal cells die, lose their nuclei and form the protective keratin of the horny layer.

Injury or removal of the upper layers of the epidermis increases the rate of mitoses in the basal layer and the gaps are repaired. Friction and the wearing away of the horny layer leads to greater production of keratin and an increased thickness. The palms and soles are a good example of this. Also situated in the basal part of the epidermis are the pigment producing cells, the melanoblasts derived from the nervous system. The dermis is composed of bundles of collagen fibres which act as a framework and support for the blood vessels, nerves, lymphatics, sweat glands and hair follicles and scattered in the dermis are histiocytes and mast cells derived from the reticulo-endothelial system.

The keratin of the epidermis is maintained supple by the secretions of the sweat and sebaceous glands and fat produced by the epidermal cells themselves. The sweat glands, which are situated deep in the der-mis, are formed of a coiled tube of cubical epithelium which leads by the sweat duct to open on the surface of the skin through spiral clefts between the epidermal cells. The sweat glands are under central nervous control and can be stimulated to secrete by the need for the body to lose heat, or by fear. Sweat is a true secretion of slightly acid pH which in general reflects the changes of the electrolytes in the plasma. The sebaceous glands are situated around and open into hair follicles. They are composed of specialised epidermal cells which form the greasy product, sebum, by the degeneration of their own cell substance in a comparable way to keratin formation by the normal epidermal cell. Sebum production is not under nervous control but is dependent on the size and mitotic activity of the sebaceous cells which are themselves influenced by the pituitary and sex hormones. The apocrine glands, which are situated in the axillae, breasts and near the genitals have features of both sweat and sebaceous glands. They are odoriferous and are a secondary sex characteristic.

Hair (See p. 171) and nails are specially modified keratin structures, both being formed by invaginations of the epidermis.

CHAPTER 3

DERMATITIS

THE epidermal cells are normally protected from damage by the
tightly packed squames of keratin of the horny layer. The elasticity
of keratin varies with its water content which can be reduced by evaporation or by removal of the lipid with which it retains moisture. Substances which produce inflammation of the epidermis (dermatitis) by
mechanical or chemical disruption of the horny layer are called primary
irritants. Degreasing agents such as soaps, if used repeatedly over a
short time will cause dryness, redness, fissuring and irritation of the
skin in almost everyone.. This traumatic or primary irritant dermatitis
which accounts for four-fifths of dermatitis in industry is not dependent on hypersensitivity or allergic reaction, although there is considerable individual variation in susceptibility. The liability to such
dermatitis will be increased in those who inherit an unduly dry skin or
in later life when the activity of the sebaceous glands declines. Thus
in old age, skin irritation may result from washing habits which in
earlier life were harmless. Normally the skin has considerable powers
of neutralising alkali but this buffering power is diminished in primary
irritant dermatitis and as a result the epidermis is more prone to damage
by alkalis.

Dermatitis or eczema

A more violent skin reaction, contact or sensitisation dermatitis may
befall the epidermis. The epidermal cells swell and disrupt, producing
a sequence of changes which appear as erythema, swelling, vesiculation
and exudation. This sequence of events, in particular the vesicular
element is termed an eczematous reaction and the confusion of terminology between dermatitis and eczema has bedevilled dermatology for
years. Eczema is a syndrome not a disease and can be caused by agents
which reach the skin from the outside surface, from the blood, or by an
inherent instability of the epidermal cells present since birth or acquired
later in life.

It has been conventional in England to call eczematous reactions
produced from outside contact dermatitis and those eruptions due to
endogenous or intrinsic factors, eczema. This arrangement has the
merit of simplicity and will be used henceforth.

**Acute contact dermatitis. (Dermatitis venenata—
Sensitisation dermatitis)**

Pathogenesis. Contact dermatitis is one of the three hypersensitivity responses shown by the skin, the others are urticaria and the delayed tuberculin reaction. Although there is hardly any substance, animal, vegetable or mineral, which cannot cause epidermal sensitivity the capacity to sensitise varies greatly. Some substances, the metal nickel for instance, produce dermatitis in a high percentage of those who handle it; other materials can be handled with impunity for many years.

The sensitiser reaches the epidermis through the horny layer, via sweat ducts and hair follicles or trivial breaks in the keratin. There it combines with protein to form a stable antigen. This then sensitises lymphocytes giving rise to a specific cell-mediated capacity to react; any further contact with the sensitiser will be followed by an explosive inflammatory reaction of the epidermis. There is always an interval between first handling a sensitiser and the development of sensitisation, which may be a few days but is usually months or years. At the time of sensitisation the whole skin of the individual becomes sensitised and experimental evidence suggests that this general sensitisation is carried on the lymphocytes. There is no circulating antibody in the serum such as is found in allergic urticaria.

Patch testing, which consists in the application of a small amount of a suspected sensitiser to an area of apparently normal skin, depends on the spread of skin sensitivity. If the test is positive, an area of dermatitis will appear beneath the patch in 24–48 hours. Because of this, contact dermatitis is sometimes called the delayed allergic reaction. If no further contact with the sensitiser occurs, there is a gradual lessening of the sensitivity but in many cases it is lifelong.

Just as the capacity of substances to sensitise varies, so the ease with which an individual can be sensitised varies. Contact dermatitis is very rare before puberty and though difficult to prove statistically, it seems to occur more often in emotional crises. A person who has reacted to one substance is more likely to develop reactions to other materials even if chemically unrelated. Sensitivities are usually specific but sometimes the body cannot distinguish between chemicals of closely related structure. Thus a patient with a dermatitis due to hair dye (paraphenylene diamine) may also be sensitive to procaine. This phenomenon, known as cross-sensitisation, may explain some of the sudden eczematous skin eruptions which arise after the first contact with a material.

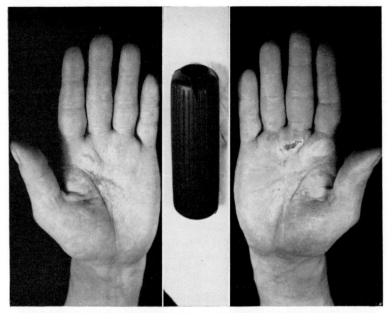

FIG. 9 (*a*).—Dermatitis of hands from handle bar grips.

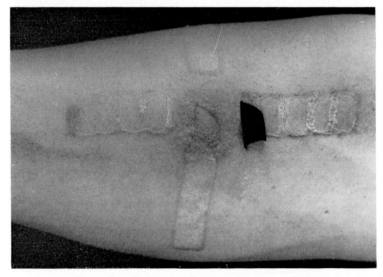

FIG. 9 (*b*).—Positive patch test in the same patient.

CLINICAL ASPECTS OF EXOGENOUS DERMATITIS

Although there is a theoretical distinction between dermatitis caused by primary irritants and true sensitisation, it may not be possible to separate the factors in an individual case. For instance, detergents remove lipid from the keratin thus allowing it to dry excessively and to split. At this stage the skin is rough and fissured, the change of a mild

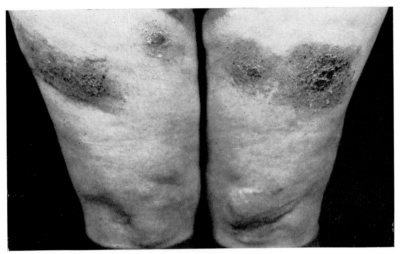

FIG. 10 (a).—Suspender dermatitis. (Nickel.)

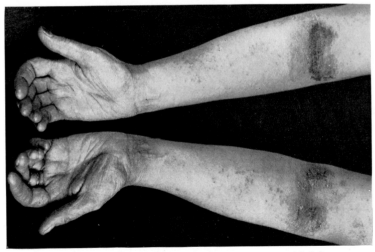

FIG. 10 (b).—Auto-sensitisation eruption in the ante cubital fossae of the same patient.

primary irritant dermatitis. The epidermal cells are now more easily damaged, since there is no longer a waterproof intact horny layer, and sensitisation of the exposed skin cells can occur as shown by an increase in the inflammatory reaction.

Although detergents have been taken as an example, other degreasing agents damage the skin in a similar way; soluble oils and even cement also do so.

Another factor which plays a significant part is mechanical trauma. Amongst women, nickel suspender dermatitis is a common problem but dermatitis frequently occurs only under the back suspender buckles, where there is more pressure and friction.

When the problem of the cause of a skin eruption is posed, the first important question to answer is whether the eruption is a dermatitis due to exogenous contact and, secondly, can it be decided whether it is a primary irritant or traumatic reaction or a specific hypersensitivity.

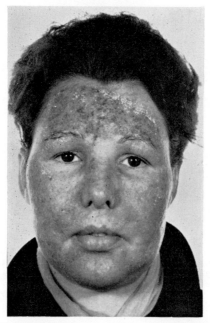

FIG. 11.—Dermatitis of the face from a rubber sponge.

The clinical features of contact dermatitis are caused by violent inflammation of the epidermis and dermis. Where the skin is loosely attached, such as around the eyelids and on the scrotum, considerable oedematous swelling may simulate urticaria or even an acute cellulitis; but vesicle formation in the epidermis, to be followed later by weeping and desquamation, should indicate dermatitis. Although the diagnosis of sensitisation dermatitis is not difficult, the identification of the sensitiser calls for detective ability.

The history is of vital importance. One is entirely dependent on the accuracy of a patient's memory for substances which have been handled but above all else it is important to determine the site of onset of the eruption since this will give a lead to the probable cause. A band of erythema around the forehead will of necessity suggest a hatband as the likely offender but contact dermatitis of the scalp caused by a hair dressing or dye will affect the skin of the forehead, ears and eyelids and may spare the scalp since this is remarkably resistant to irritants of all kinds.

The eyelids are susceptible indicators of sensitivity and may be involved in dermatitis from dusts, vapours and cosmetics. A common

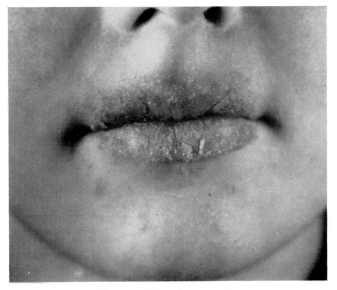

FIG. 12.—Lipstick dermatitis.

catch for the unwary is the dermatitis of eyelids produced by nail varnish. Since the varnish is applied to the inert nail-plate no change can be seen on the fingers but isolated areas on the side of the neck and lids may be involved by occasional contact with the varnished nails.

Face powder, cream, rouge and lipstick all can produce dermatitis limited to the face and do not be misled by the patient who stoutly maintains that she has used the same brand for years. She may have taken years to become sensitive, or, a point that is often overlooked, the makers may have altered the constituents. Chemicals which may be light sensitisers are often added to soap and toilet preparations. Such photosensitive eruptions affect the face, V of the neck and the exposed parts of the limbs.

A knowledge of the habits of men and women is necessary to pose the right questions. Dermatitis behind the ears due to nylon hair-nets worn at night and dermatitis of the cheeks due to rubber sponges used for applying liquid make-up, are two examples which require some inside knowledge to elicit the cause.

Sensitivity to various articles of clothing can be diagnosed by the characteristic pattern of involvement. Ties produce a localised area at the front of the neck and beneath the chin. Shirts involve the axillary folds, the sides of the neck and the buttocks and thighs in those who wear their shirts beneath their pants.

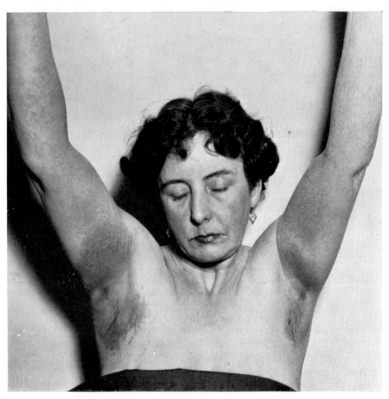

FIG. 13.—Clothing dermatitis which spares the apices of
the axillae.

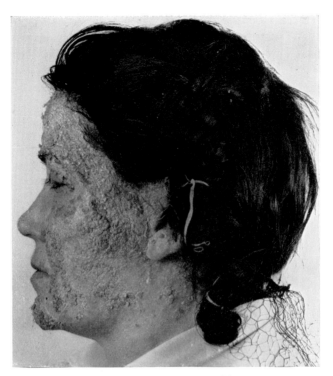

FIG. 14.—Hair dye dermatitis.

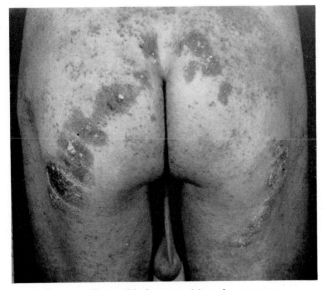

FIG. 15.—Dermatitis from varnish on lavatory seat.

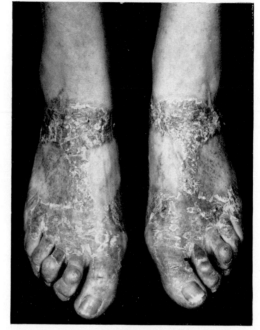

Fig. 16.—Shoe dermatitis.

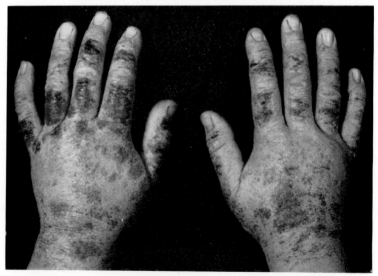

Fig. 17.—Contact dermatitis of hands from industrial gloves.

The axillary lesions affect only the anterior and posterior folds, sparing the apex which does not touch the clothing. This is a useful differential diagnostic point, since the endogenous eruptions of psoriasis and seborrhoeic eczema involve the whole axilla.

Do not forget that dyes are not the only possible offenders in clothing. Formalin used in some drip-dry clothing, and other chemical finishes and even the man-made fibres themselves which may be colourless, can cause dermatitis.

A regional grouping of likely causes can be made—

Scalp. Hair dyes, brilliantines and scalp lotions.

Ears. May be involved by scalp applications, but also hair-nets, spectacle frames, ear clips, hearing aids and ear drops.

Eyelids and face. Plant sensitivity, airborne dusts, volatile chemicals, cosmetics, soap and nail varnish.

Neck. Ties, scarves, furs, necklaces (particularly the nickel and chrome clasps), nail varnish (from the habit of resting the chin in the hand), perfume.

Axillae. Clothing, rubber arm shields, deodorants.

Trunk. Clothing, rubber and synthetic elastic undergarments.

Perianal region. Local application and toilet papers, lavatory seat.

Genitals. Dusts, clothing, contraceptives.

Thighs. Suspenders, either nickel or chromium and rubber, articles carried in pockets, matchboxes, chrome-plated objects.

Ankles and feet. Socks, stockings, rubber and metal foot supports, chemical dusts, rubber boots and shoes, dyes and adhesives used in shoe manufacture.

Hands and forearms. Innumerable materials handled at work or in the house (liquids will tend to affect the finger webs and backs of the fingers and hands rather than the palms), plant sensitivity, rubber gloves and finger stalls, (palmar lesions are rare, but may occur from gripping tool handles, car gear levers, plastic, or rubber cycle grips, racket and club handles.)

Primula sensitivity

Though a wide range of plants can produce contact dermatitis the common cause in Britain is *primula obconica*, the indoor primula. This causes a violent vesicular eruption on the fingers and forearms with the usual linear distribution of plant reactions due to contact with the leaves, and an urticarial swelling of the face and neck. This curious mixture of urticaria and dermatitis is not seen in other plant reactions. The degree of sensitivity may be so great that patients can diagnose the presence of a primula plant, probably hidden behind a curtain, by the onset of itching.

Dermatitis from other plants such as chrysanthemums, the next most common cause, is a less violent eruption which because of the

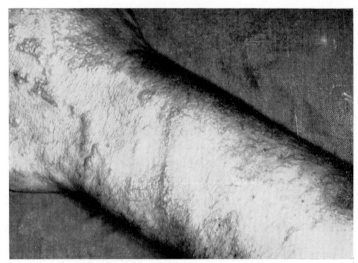

FIG. 18.—Primula sensitivity. Note linear blisters.

redness and lichenification on the face and hands resembles atopic
eczema.

A rare source of severe blistering on the exposed skin is contact with
a plant which produces photosensitivity and this explanation should
be suspected in agricultural workers (from handling parsnips) and
picnickers who may lie on the stinking mayweed (anthemis) or
gardeners cutting down the giant hogweed.

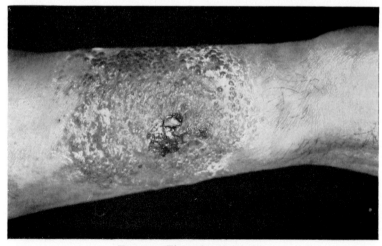

FIG. 19.—Elastoplast dermatitis.

Medicaments applied to the skin are a common cause of sensitisation dermatitis and almost every application is capable of sensitising some-one. A trivial abrasion can be converted into a violent weeping derma-titis by the use of a household antiseptic. Eyedrops, eardrops, rubbing oils, plasters are all potential causes of dermatitis. In a survey of over 100 proven examples of dermatitis caused by medicaments, antibiotics,

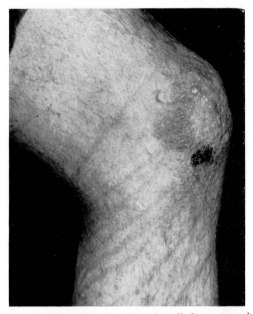

FIG. 20.—Dermatitis from Dettol applied to a wound.

local anaesthetic ointments and locally applied antihistamine prepar-ations were the most common offenders. There is in our opinion no justification for the use of penicillin, sulphonamides, chloramphenicol, benzocaine and the other "cain" anaesthetics or antihistamines as local applications. Neomycin has been widely condemned as a common cause of dermatitis but it has been used more extensively than most other antibiotics and in our view the danger has possibly been exag-gerated. The ointment bases including lanolin and the antiseptics (parabens) used to prevent bacterial contamination of ointments may cause sensitisation. Such a happening can explain aggravation of skin disorders by topical steroid applications which should in theory lessen inflammation. Sensitivities to medicaments arise most frequently around varicose dermatitis in leg ulcers, probably because of the long continued duration of treatment in these areas.

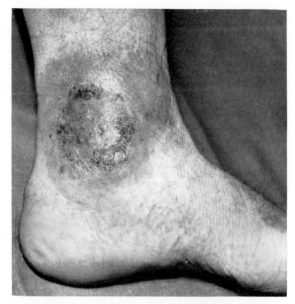

FIG. 21 (*a*).—Dermatitis from medicament applied to gravitational ulcer.

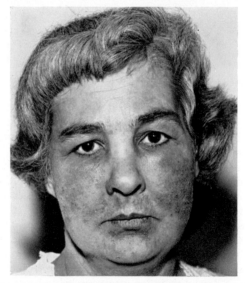

FIG. 21 (*b*).—Auto-sensitisation eruption of the face in the same patient.

The Patch Test

The identification of the exact cause of dermatitis can often be made by patch tests. We prefer to narrow the list of suspected substances by careful history taking but in some centres, notably in Scandinavia, tests are carried out on every patient with a battery of common sensitisers. Whilst some unexpected positive reactions are discovered there is a risk of sensitising patients by patch tests.

Patch tests should not be performed whilst dermatitis is acute as this may be aggravated by the further slight contact with the sensitiser.

A small portion of the suspected material is applied to an area of skin not involved by the dermatitis, usually the back or the outer aspects of the arm. If a fluid is being tested it is adsorbed on a square of gauze. This is then covered with cellophane or some other inert impermeable material. A ready prepared strip of aluminium foil such as Al test is useful. The whole is held in position with adhesive tape. Control tests with similar materials should also be applied. If a patient is known to have a sensitivity to adhesive strapping the "patches" can be held in position by proprietary tapes such as Blenderm, Dermicel or Micropore which are less irritant than the commonly used Elasto-patches. The tests are left in position for 48 hours unless the discomfort of a violently positive reaction demands an earlier removal. A positive reaction consists of an area of inflammation beneath the suspected material which may vary from mild erythema to vesiculation or rarely necrosis. It is wise to wait 10 to 20 minutes after the patch has been removed since oedema may be suppressed by the pressure of the patch. If negative, the site of the patch should be inspected again 2 days later. Very mild but positive reactions are slow in appearing. Care should be taken in interpreting results of tests. False positives may be due to using test materials which are in themselves primary irritants or, if the dermatitis is still active, a non specific false positive may be produced by the slight trauma of the test. A negative test does not exclude the substance as the cause of the dermatitis because the exact conditions under which it has been handled may not have been reproduced. Volatile substances such as perfumes which cause primary irritation under occlusion can be painted on the skin as an open patch test. Photocontact allergy must be confirmed by photo-patch testing. Paired patch tests are applied for 24 hours. Then one series of the test patches are removed and the areas irradiated with ultra violet light. Photosensitivity is shown by a positive response 24–48 hours later on the irradiated test areas.

A usage test, i.e. further handling of the substance under natural conditions when the dermatitis has recovered may be the only way to prove the diagnosis if patch tests are negative.

2

Some substances give positive patch tests only if the horny layer has previously been stripped off the site. Neomycin sensitivity can be demonstrated in this way and other medicaments such as the antihistamines also need a stripped skin test to confirm the sensitivity.

DISSEMINATION OF CONTACT DERMATITIS

After an area of contact dermatitis has existed for some time (the period may vary from days to months), extension to other parts of the body often occurs. This has been explained by the theory that some product of damaged skin, either alone or with bacteria, produces specific antibodies. Once these are present in sufficient amount, extension of the dermatitis to other areas of the skin will occur. This theory of auto-sensitisation is an attractive one, but as yet remains unproved.

There is a very definite pattern of spread from initial sites. For instance, lesions on the hands will first extend to the feet and vice versa. Lesions of the legs produce eruptions on the opposite leg and then on the forearms, face and neck.

Dermatitis of the scalp will involve the other hairy areas, the axillae and groins.

Occasionally the signs of this secondary dermatitis are more obvious than the primary lesion. Thus, swelling and itching of the eyelids and the hands may worry the patient more than small patches of suspender dermatitis on the legs, which unless searched for, will be missed.

Another common occurrence is generalised spread from a varicose dermatitis of the leg aggravated by a medicament. Once this generalised spread has occurred, the skin remains in an excitable state. Any further skin damage, even years later, may precipitate a recurrence of generalised dermatitis.

Very occasionally the state of generalised exfoliative dermatitis can be initiated by exogenous causes. In this condition the whole of the skin surface becomes involved in an angry erythema with constant shedding of scales followed in many cases by the loss of hair and nails.

TREATMENT OF CONTACT DERMATITIS

Identification and removal of the exciting cause is the first step in treatment. The nature of the disorder should be explained to the patient since fear and anxiety will aggravate symptoms. The avoidance of skin irritants such as disinfectants and strong soaps should be stressed, and the technique of treatment to be used carefully explained to the patient.

Local treatment of acute dermatitis. The aim of local treatment is to relieve discomfort and prevent further damage to the epidermis. This has traditionally been achieved by cooling the hot inflamed skin by evaporation from wet dressings of inert lotions such as calamine lotion B.P. Such treatment requires considerable nursing skill and the dampness may add to the patient's discomfort. An application of one of the anti-inflammatory topical corticosteroids is now the usual first choice of treatment for the ambulant patient.

Corticosteroids are prescribable in three main vehicles, lotions, ointments and creams, and an aerosol spray. Lotions are preferable for acute exuding lesions, creams or ointments should be used for less inflamed dry skin. There is no indication for aerosol sprays which are wasteful and the drying of the skin caused by the volatile vehicle may be uncomfortable. Lotions should be applied by squeezing a small amount from the plastic bottle on to the finger protected by a disposable finger stall. The lotion should be spread as thinly as possible. The fact that the area is moist with serum is no bar to this method but adjacent skin surfaces which may become adherent should be separated by a layer of linen or gauze. No covering is needed for the face and other exposed areas but patients may feel more comfortable if the limbs are covered by Tubegauze and the hands by cotton gloves. Applications should be repeated 6–8 times daily and reduced in frequency as the inflammation lessens. Sudden cessation of treatment should be avoided as a rebound acute recurrence of the dermatitis may follow. The corticosteroid applications must be gradually tailed off to once daily, alternate days and even twice weekly. It has been shown that a reservoir of steroid remains under the horny layer for as long as a week and small amounts continue to be released to the underlying dermis.

All the corticosteroids reduce erythema, oedema and exudation and in the treatment of acute dermatitis hydrocortisone, the first to be introduced, is almost as effective as the modern more actively penetrating preparations. The main disadvantage of the powerful steroids such as fluocinolone (Synalar) and betamethasone (Betnovate) in their standard strengths is their ability to damage the collagen of the dermis producing temporary atrophy. They should therefore be used as sparingly as possible, and avoided particularly on the face, and in the axillae and groins, where telangiectases and striae may be quickly produced. They can be used safely in a dilution of 1 in 10 in a cream base when their activity is roughly comparable to that of 1% hydrocortisone. The indication for their use in standard strength is in the treatment of hands and feet where hydrocortisone is less effective as it cannot penetrate the thick skin. Acute dermatitis of the hands and feet should therefore be treated with betamethasone (Betnovate) or fluocinolone (Synalar) or other similar steroids. If there is not a speedy response then extra penetration may be attained by occlusion for 8 hours nightly under plastic gloves or bags.

Normally no antiseptic or antibiotic need be combined with the steroid and, in fact, they are better avoided as they may sensitise the already inflamed skin. For the same reason antihistamine preparations, in particular those mixed with calamine, should not be used. The only exception for combining an antiseptic effective against candida with a steroid is when treating such areas as the perianal region or the external ear.

Areas of dermatitis should not be washed with soap but should be cleaned with an emulsion of water and ung. emulsificans, liquid paraffin or olive oil.

In very severe and extensive cases of dermatitis which require hospital admission a combination of topical steroid and treatment with wet dressings is often most comforting to the patient. A steroid lotion is applied first and then the area covered with linen which has been soaked in calamine lotion, and all skin surfaces which come in contact with each other separated by layers of linen. The dressings may be held in position by Tubegauze or Netalast. Such wet dressings must be changed before they have dried but this is well-nigh impracticable during the night and an alternative is to permit the patient to moisten the dressings from the outside with more lotion. After a night's sleep (a patient should not be awakened for dressings) the linen is likely to be adherent to exuding areas. Soaking the adherent linen with more lotion for some 10 minutes before the re-dressing is carried out will assist removal without damage to the epidermis.

Where secondary infection is obvious particularly in treating hands and feet, wet dressings of $\frac{1}{4}$ strength Sodium Hypochlorite Solution Dilute B.P.C. (Milton) are effective and infection should also be controlled by systemic antibiotics. Rest in bed lowers capillary pressure in both upper and lower limbs and will assist the control of persistent exudation.

Treatment of sub-acute and chronic dermatitis. When a dermatitis has persisted for some time the skin becomes thick, scaly and lichenified and the habit of scratching is deeply ingrained. The addition of an antipruritic such as coal tar to compound zinc paste may lessen skin damage and allow healing to occur. Often it may be necessary to use an occlusive medicated bandage which can be applied directly to the skin and kept in position for 7 days. These can be applied to fingers separately, held in position by Tubegauze, thus allowing a dry hand occupation to be continued. Bandages are impregnated with simple zinc paste, ichthyol paste, coal tar paste and even corticosteroids. Coal tar bandages have in our hands been most effective in chronic dermatitis. The great advantage of occlusion is that anxiety is lessened by hiding the lesions, experiments in self-treatment are impossible and injury from scratching is cut to a minimum. In resistant dermatitis, particularly of the hands and feet, the application of the fluocinolone or similar corticosteroid beneath an occlusive polythene covering may cure where all else has failed (see appendix).

Drugs. There is no specific internal remedy for dermatitis but in some cases there is an undoubted dermal component or urticarial element responsible for itching which can be controlled by antihistamine drugs. Since the majority of antihistamines also have a sedative effect this is also of benefit. Promethazine hydrochloride (Phenergan) 50 mg. at night or chlorpromazine hydrochloride (Largactil) 25 mg. in the morning and 50 mg. at night in the elderly are effective. A good night's sleep is vitally important and of the sedatives dichloralphenazone (Welldorm) or nitrazepam (Mogadon) are safe and effective.

There is a temptation to use systemic corticosteroids in widespread dermatitis. This should be resisted in all but the very worst situations for although symptoms may be suppressed by corticosteroids there is often considerable difficulty in the withdrawal of treatment without recurrence of the eruption. Should the decision be made to use corticosteroids then prednisolone 10 mg. three times a day is a standard starting dosage, which should be lowered as soon as the skin shows improvement. One absolute indication for the use of corticosteroids would be the onset of true exfoliative dermatitis.

Light dermatitis

The possible diagnosis of light sensitisation of the skin should arise if an erythematous or vesicular eruption appears on the areas of the face, neck and hands which are normally exposed to sunlight. The parts involved resemble those affected in a dust dermatitis but light eruptions spare the eyelids, the upper lip and the neck under the chin as all these regions are in shadow. A helpful point in the history will be the seasonal variation; in Britain most light eruptions begin in the spring—March or April—and clear at the end of September.

Light reactions have been divided into phototoxic in which there is an exaggerated sunburn response which soon passes off and photo-allergic which once induced may persist for years.

The causes of photosensitive reactions are similar to the causes of any eczematous eruption. Thus photosensitivity can occur from external contact sensitisers, from drugs and metabolites and as a spontaneous disorder comparable to constitutional eczema. Eosin in lipstick, perfumes in cosmetics and pitch and tar fumes are well known contact light sensitisers and in recent years a germicide added to a popular soap produced an "epidemic" of photosensitisation. Most chemical causes of light eruptions are themselves "fluorescent".

A very wide range of drugs produce light sensitivity and the possibility should be considered in any light eruption. Of those in popular use the phenothiazines, sulphonamides, chlorothiazides and demethyl chlortetracycline head the list. Some produce light sensitivity when used as local medicaments as well as when taken internally. Confirmation of the diagnosis can be obtained by photo-patch testing (see page 25).

Polymorphic light eruptions

In many light eruptions a sensitising chemical either of exogenous or endogenous origin cannot be found. Such eruptions may appear rarely as bullae on the face in childhood and more commonly as a papular eruption on the upper margin of the ears in early spring. In adults an idiopathic light eruption often starts after severe sunburn. The following spring an irritable eruption of papules, plaques and vesicles appears and persists throughout the summer months. Often this will recur year after year in the same month, clearing in the autumn. There may be difficulty in differentiating such eruptions from discoid lupus erythematosus or from disseminated lupus erythematosus, and an apparently benign light eruption may after some years show the biochemical change of lupus erythematosus. It is most important therefore that idiopathic light eruption be investigated thoroughly to exclude both lupus erythematosus (see page 118) or porphyria (see page 199) which can also produce light sensitivity.

Treatment. The immediate treatment is that of any dermatitis. The skin may be protected against further exposure by applying creams which either prevent the passage of light rays by their content of opaque powder such as titanium dioxide or by their ability to absorb the wavelength which damages the skin, usually 290 to 320 nm. Mexenone (Uvistat) is a popular and effective light-absorbent cream. It can be combined if necessary with an opaque powder if it is not effective alone.

Antimalarial drugs, such as Chloroquin sulphate 200 mg. daily, do alleviate some cases of light sensitivity but, in view of the side effects, should be used for only very short periods such as the 2 to 3 weeks of a summer holiday. There are a number of sufferers from a light eruption who cannot be relieved by medicaments and for them shady hats, long sleeves and gloves remain an uncomfortable solution.

CHAPTER 4

INDUSTRIAL DERMATITIS

OCCUPATIONAL or industrial dermatitis does not differ from exogenous dermatitis previously described except for the circumstances of its onset. In the National Insurance Act, Prescribed Disease 42 is defined as non-infective dermatitis caused wholly or partly by contact with dust, liquid or vapour or any other skin irritant encountered at work.

(i) *Traumatic dermatitis.* Some 70 per cent of industrial dermatitis is caused by direct damage to the epidermis by friction from abrasive dust such as coal, stone or brick, or glass wool or the effect of primary irritants. Primary irritants include acids, alkalis and chemicals which when in contact with the skin for a sufficient time in adequate concentration produce cell damage. Included in this group are the simple alkaline degreasing agents such as soap and water or brine and the soluble oils or coolants used widely in the engineering industry. The more searching solvents like paraffin, petroleum and carbon tetrachloride, white spirit, paint thinners and turpentine are even more potent causes of skin damage.

(ii) *Sensitisation or contact dermatitis.* Many of the substances handled in industry like those in the home are sensitisers, but only a small proportion of workers at risk develop dermatitis and sensitisation is responsible for only 14 per cent of industrial dermatitis. Common examples are the epoxy resins used to join materials in numerous light industries, nickel and chrome solutions, dyes, photographic chemicals and sawdust from hardwoods such as teak, iroko or rosewood. Some primary irritants, such as the soluble oils, may at times act as sensitisers and they often contain substances such as antiseptics which are more liable to cause sensitisation than the oil itself.

(iii) *The tired skin.* After many years of wear and tear of the skin by very mild irritant dusts or liquids, dermatitis may develop. This is seen commonly in the elderly coal miner or building trade worker.

(iv) *Constitutional eczema aggravated by exogenous irritants.* An individual who is eczema prone is more likely to develop an exacerbation of eczema if exposed to working conditions which are unsuitable. It may be extremely difficult to decide what part has been played by exogenous irritants and such cases are often the subject of litigation. It can be argued that anyone who develops a dermatitis in conditions which do not harm the majority of his workmates, has a constitutional weakness of the skin and in support of this is the finding that the age distribution of coal miners with exogenous dermatitis was similar to

31

that of coal miners considered to have endogenous eczema. Only after observation over a period of years may it be possible in an individual case to assess correctly the relative importance of exogenous irritants and constitutional weakness.

DIAGNOSIS OF INDUSTRIAL DERMATITIS

It must be established that the skin lesion was not present before the worker started the occupation. The exact nature of the work must be known and this may entail a visit to the factory. Any recent change in working methods and materials should be sought. A recent injury to the skin may predispose the worker to an attack of dermatitis and in many cases the dermatitis may be due to antiseptics applied to a wound. A history of improvement at weekends and gradual recurrence during the week is suggestive and sensitisation sometimes starts after a holiday because some degree of immunity is lost.

The skin eruption usually begins in those areas most exposed to possible irritants. The hands and forearms are therefore the common sites and in right handed workers the right hand is more severely involved. The sides and backs of the fingers, the webs between and the front of the wrists are affected more than the palms whose thick horny layer acts as a protection. Primary irritant dermatitis due to solvents often starts beneath wedding or signet rings which prevent the finger being adequately washed and dried. Where a volatile substance is the cause the initial site may be the eyelids, face and neck. Dusts cling to moist skin and the axillae, groins and scrotum may be the initial sites affected. It should not be forgotten that cleansing agents and even protective clothing, gloves and barrier creams may cause dermatitis. Often the habit of rinsing the hands in a solvent to remove grease causes more damage than the long contact with oils throughout the working day and dermatitis caused by rubber gloves may complicate a simple traumatic dermatitis.

It is to be expected that industrial dermatitis should improve if work is stopped but in very chronic cases where the eruption has persisted for some years a state of eczema develops in which new lesions erupt without further contact with irritants. Here again the distinction between exogenous dermatitis and endogenous factors may be well nigh impossible. Once the skin defences have been broken down, non-specific irritants such as heat, friction and washing can maintain the skin inflammation.

Special types of industrial skin disease

Dermatitis may follow injury and this should be distinguished from the usual prescribed disease. The dermatitis may be an infective eczematoid reaction after a cut or burn, or more frequently the result of the application of a sensitising local antiseptic to a wound. The patient can be reassured that it will be safe to return to his usual occupation since it was the wound and not the job which was responsible for the dermatitis.

(i) **Industrial acne.** A follicular pustular reaction on the face, trunk and limbs is produced by exposure to vapours of chlorinated naphthalenes used in insulating cable. Similar lesions can be caused by coal tar and pitch but the most frequent cause is contact with insoluble cutting oils of high boiling point. These produce thickening of the keratin at the opening of the hair follicles which results in blackhead and pustule formation most commonly on the forearms and thighs. There is considerable individual variation in susceptibility and oil acne is more likely to develop in the young inexpert worker whose boiler suit becomes soaked in oil.

(ii) **Chrome ulcers.** Ulceration of the skin of the fingers and the nasal septum occurs in those exposed to chromic acid and chromates. The ulcer forms around trivial abrasions.

(iii) **Occupational cancer.** The substances which produce keratin change in the epidermis can over a period of years act as carcinogens. At first simple keratoses or warts, which are non-malignant, form, but true epitheliomatous change eventually occurs possibly years after exposure to the carcinogen. Tar, pitch, bitumen and the mineral oils are the main offenders and lesions appear usually on the exposed skin but an additional classical site is the scrotum. Contact with pitch occurs in some unlikely trades, for instance optical lens polishing and an industrial origin should be sought for all warty lesions on the skin.

(iv) **Skin damage from radiation.** An increasing hazard is exposure to radio-active materials and X-rays which can produce an acute burn followed by a necrosis and ulceration or a chronic dermatitis with atrophy telangiectasis and cracking. Malignant change may complicate the chronic radiation damage.

Epidermophytosis. It has been accepted in the coal mining industry that fungus infection of the toes is an occupational hazard and this is spread by the pithead baths. It affects up to 50 per cent of coal miners in some pits. The Ministry of Health and Social Security recognise this disease when it affects colliers and it is classed as an industrial injury.

PREVENTION

The prevention of dermatitis in industry depends on several factors, selection of personnel, protection, cleanliness and education of the workmen. Although it is recognised that dark skinned workers are less susceptible to sensitisers and degreasing agents than fair skinned but more prone to folliculitis, it is seldom practicable to select employees on this basis. An attempt should be made to exclude from contact with degreasing agents those with dry ichthyotic skins and exclude from hot dusty surroundings the worker who has a previous history of atopic or seborrhoeic eczema.

PROTECTION

As far as possible, workers should not be required to handle either primary irritants or sensitisers and to bring this about it may be necessary to redesign machinery. Substances which are known causes of dermatitis should be eliminated, for example the inclusion of antiseptics in coolants. There is little need for these to prevent infection, but they increase the risk of dermatitis. Where some contact cannot be avoided, protective clothing, aprons, boots and gloves should be worn. Rubber or polythene gloves may cause maceration of the skin if worn for long periods. This can be prevented by wearing absorbent inner gloves. Boiler suits which are contaminated with oil or dust should be cleaned regularly. Numerous creams designed to be applied before work and to form a protective coating have been devised and yet there is no effective barrier cream, and a belief in the effectiveness may lead to the neglect of other more important steps in the prevention of dermatitis. The main virtue of barrier creams is in facilitating the removal of dirt and in reducing the trauma to the skin from scrubbing brushes, abrasives and soaps. Of more value in the reduction of dermatitis is the introduction of effective and safe cleansing agents such as the sulphonated oils and better facilities for washing at work.

Adequate discussion of the causes and prevention of dermatitis are helpful since neither worker nor manager will co-operate in preventive measures unless the need is understood. There is still a belief that dermatitis is contagious and that it carries a social stigma and this idea should be combated vigorously on the shop floor and in the board-room.

TREATMENT OF INDUSTRIAL DERMATITIS

In general the patient should cease contact with the cause of dermatitis though in a few cases such as in the explosives industry desensitisation or hardening occurs if the worker continues in the same job with less exposure. This is a rare phenomenon. The usual course of events is for the dermatitis to become worse if further contact is not prevented. This does not imply that the worker should cease work but he should be moved to some other job. The use of occlusive dressings should enable suitable dry hand work to be continued. It is much more difficult to resettle a man once he has been out of work, and the anxiety about his future aggravates the skin condition. Change of occupation must be permanent for patients with sensitisation dermatitis as relapse speedily follows even slight contact with the offending agent. In traumatic dermatitis, return to the original job may be possible if provision is made for increased protection against the irritant. It has been found however that the relapse rate in traumatic dermatitis is far higher than in sensitisation dermatitis where the worker has been moved from the sensitiser. It has been our experience that workers of good morale settle themselves without assistance. Those who need aid are the elderly with the tired skin syndrome who have difficulty in finding a job. The individual with an inadequate personality cannot deal with the situation when he develops dermatitis and the patient who has had a long period off work becomes discouraged. They both need rehabilitation. The disabled persons' register is of no value to patients with dermatitis because employers will not accept a known sufferer from dermatitis.

CHAPTER 5

ECZEMA

BY definition eczema means an itching vesicular skin eruption and some dermatologists include in this group all diseases which have the eczema reaction in the epidermis; this would include contact dermatitis and eczematous reactions caused by exogenous irritants.

A more practical working arrangement is to accept within the diagnosis eczematous vesicular eruptions for which there is no apparent external cause.

The mechanism of auto-sensitisation in which lesions arise far from the primary area of inflammation illustrates the possibility of eruptions arising from an endogenous source and it is well recognised that any widespread eruption, even of exogenous origin, can become chronic and fresh lesions arise without any further contact with the irritant. This persistence of irritable weeping patches with recurrent and sporadic outbreaks of new lesions is characteristic of the state of eczema. It may well be that damage to skin cells by scratching releases an antigen which in turn causes further epidermal destruction and the condition is self perpetuating. It can be seen therefore that without an adequate history it may be impossible to distinguish from the clinical appearance of one group of eczematous lesions whether the disease is of exogenous or endogenous origin. Indeed there are endogenous or constitutional factors in all patients who have eczema or dermatitis but in those who suffer from eczema the constitutional tendency is the more important. With increasing knowledge and the identification of more exogenous sensitisers, the eczema group has diminished but there still remain a number of recognisable clinical varieties of constitutional or endogenous eczema.

Nummular eczema (Discoid eczema)

This term is given to coin shaped, clear cut discs of erythema surmounted by vesicles and crusts which occur mainly on the limbs. It is rare in childhood but its incidence increases rapidly in adolescence, particularly in girls. Irritation is usually intense when fresh vesicles are erupting. The common mode of onset is on the backs of the hands and fingers when a girl first does manual work. Skin trauma plays some part as protective occlusive dressings often heal the lesions which recur as soon as the bandages are removed. Nummular eczema may also arise as a pattern of auto-sensitisation from a patch of chronic stasis eczema.

In middle aged men it can erupt quite suddenly without a primary
lesion and seems in this group to be associated with emotional tension.
In men aged 60 to 65 nummular patches often appear first on the fronts
of the legs. There it occurs on the slightly ichthyotic skin over the
shins, where the first signs of failure of sebaceous glands and conse-
quent degreasing of the skin appear. Too frequent bathing has an

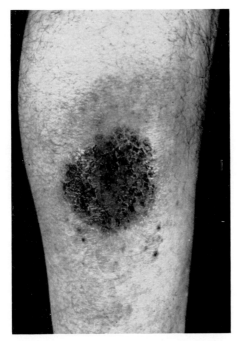

FIG. 22.—Nummular eczema.

aggravating effect in the elderly and improvement may result in a
reduction in the use of soap.

The presence of vesicles and clear cut inflamed discs should make
possible its differentiation with psoriasis. Prognosis in nummular
eczema is not good. A high percentage of 500 patients examined at the
Royal Infirmary, Sheffield five years after their initial attack still had
active eczema.

Treatment. Unlike most eczematous eruptions, topical corticosteroid preparations are not particularly effective, whereas lotions and
pastes containing tar are useful. Occlusive tar bandages applied to
fingers and hands may enable a dry hand job to be continued whilst the
eczema recovers. The bandages should be changed weekly and a light

smear of Zinc and Salicylic Acid Paste B.P. with 1% Crude coal tar
substituted in the healing stages. In the elderly, liquor picis carbonis
3% in aqueous cream B.P. or Boots E. 45 cream provides a clean
application which also adds some grease to the skin.

Infective eczema

A trivial burn or cut may be complicated by the onset of a weeping,
vesicular eruption which rapidly spreads to the surrounding skin.
Though sensitivity to an antiseptic is often the cause, eczematous
eruptions do arise where no medicament has been applied. A similar
condition occurs beneath plaster of Paris bandages where trivial skin
infection or injury has been covered. On the palm of the hand the manner

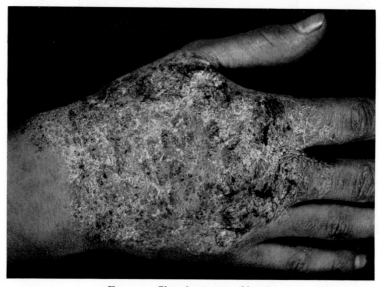

Fig. 23.—Chronic eczema of hand.

in which the clear cut undermined edge slowly extends with a fresh
crop of vesicles resembles a fungus infection, but no such organism
can be found. Pyogenic bacteria can be cultured readily and it has been
suggested that the epidermis has been sensitised to the organisms,
though this has never been confirmed experimentally.

Treatment. Reactions to medicaments are easily produced in these
cases and a generalised dissemination of the eruption is a frequent
complication. Combination of corticosteroid with an antibiotic may be
effective but failures do occur and, if so, wet dressings of ¼ strength
Sodium Hypochlorite Dilute B.P.C. (Milton) or ½% silver nitrate are

effective and safe. Systemic antibiotics may occasionally be needed to control the spread of the eruption. For local application to the generalised eruption, calamine or terra silica lotion containing $\frac{1}{4}\%$ crude coal tar is often more successful than the more modern preparations, or lotions without tar. Hospitalisation may be necessary for severe cases and is to be preferred to the giving of systemic corticosteroids, since such patients are difficult to wean off steroids.

Lichenification (Lichen simplex)

When inflamed and particularly eczematous skin is exposed to prolonged scratching, normal skin markings are exaggerated and an

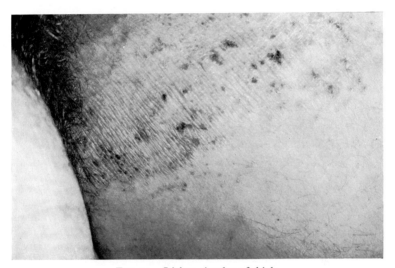

FIG. 24.—Lichen simplex of thigh.

appearance resembling morocco leather develops. This thickening takes the form of a sheet or plaque and it can be distinguished from the disease lichen planus by the absence of outlying individual papules. Lichenification merely indicates that the patient is scratching.

Some areas on the body are more liable than others to be scratched. The nape of the neck in women and the perianal region and scrotum in men are common sites for lichen simplex. An alternative name for the condition is localised neurodermatitis since it is recognised that most patients who suffer from this are tense, excitable people and the urge to scratch is more a bad habit allied to nail biting than a disease. A vicious circle of irritation, scratching, lichenification, more irritation is set up.

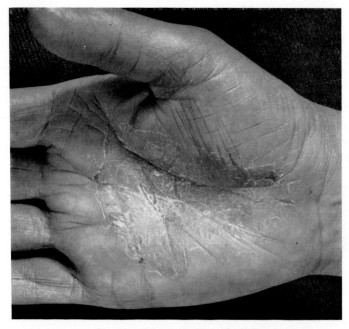

FIG. 25.—Lichen simplex of palm.

Treatment. Although it may be possible to protect the patient from further skin damage by occlusive dressings or relieve the irritation by the application of a topical corticosteroid cream, it is important to discover why the patient has lichen simplex. The skin irritation may be an outlet for an impossible life situation and removal of the method of emotional release without full discussion may in fact be harmful. Suboccipital lichen simplex may complicate psoriasis of the scalp and failure to relieve the itching may be due to the underlying psoriasis which will need its appropriate treatment.

Chronic eczema of the palms and soles

Patients who suffer from recurrent attacks of irritable vesicles in the thickened skin of the palms and soles are a common problem. Because the vesicles are under a thickened horny layer their appearance, like sago grains, differs somewhat from eczema elsewhere and names such as cheiropompholyx and dyshidrotic eczema have been coined in the belief that the vesicles were due to a disorder of the sweat apparatus.

It is probable that the majority of such cases are merely examples of chronic eczema in a special site.

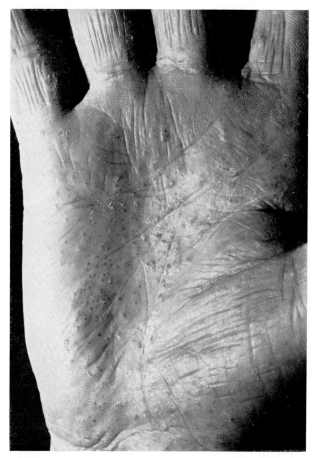

FIG. 26.—Chronic eczema of palm.

Undoubtedly some cases are due to contact sensitivities, others are eruptions secondary to fungus infections of the feet, a few are due to sensitivity to foods and drugs but in a large percentage, however carefully they are investigated, no identifiable cause can be found.

When faced with a chronic eruption of the hands and feet the following questions must be answered:

(1) Is the eruption an eczematous one?

(2) Is the major cause exogenous or endogenous?

(3) If exogenous is it due to a primary irritant or a sensitiser?

(4) Is there active fungus infection of the feet?

There is in the "idiopathic" eczemas a common association with emotional stress and this aspect is worth investigation.

Treatment. Many of the mild cases require only an emollient cream such as aqueous cream B.P. together with sedation. If pyogenic infection complicates the condition, then wet compresses of hypochlorite solution and a systemic antibiotic may be required. Topical steroids with polythene occlusion offer the best means of control but patients soon tire of the need to apply these dressings each night. Occlusive Coltapaste bandages are often of value when the steroids fail.

Atopic eczema (Infantile eczema)

Atopic eczema occurs as a clear cut entity and from the history alone it should be possible to be distinguished from other skin disorders.

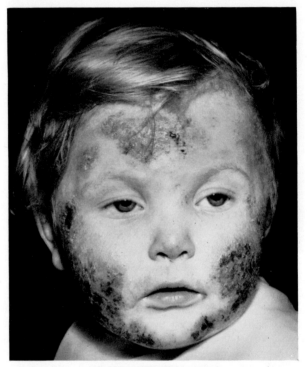

FIG. 27.—Infantile eczema.

The name atopy denotes an inherited predisposition to asthma, hay fever and eczema. The incidence in the general population has never been assessed but in one survey of infants, 3 per cent had a moderate amount of eczema and it was considered that mild degrees of eczema were even more common. Respiratory symptoms of hay fever and asthma may develop later in life or at the same time as the eczema and exacerbation of the skin and respiratory symptoms may occur together or, more frequently, as one improves the other worsens. A family history of eczema, asthma or hay fever is present in 70 per cent. Both sufferers from atopic eczema and a high percentage of their relatives give positive reactions to intracutaneous tests with protein such as egg albumen, moulds and pollens. This is a result of an inherited non-specific reactivity and is accompanied by an increase in immunoglobulins IgE and IgG and an associated lowered resistance to viral infections. The skin capillaries also react to stimulation in an abnormal manner. Light firm pressure gives rise to prolonged capillary contraction, a phenomenon called white dermographism.

In some children the eczema tendency is inherited with another genetic defect, ichthyosis. Thus even when the eczema is quiescent, the dry scaly skin of the ichthyotic is still a problem.

Clinical features. Eczema starts in infants, hence the name infantile eczema, at about the third or fourth month. Redness and scaling appear on the scalp around the cradle cap and soon spread to the cheeks. Groups of itchy red papules erupt and weep. Often the child is too young to scratch but will rub its head and face on the pillow. The eruption, in severe cases, spreads to the limbs and napkin area and because of the discomfort the child does not sleep and will keep its parents awake by crying. In severe cases, almost the whole body surface is involved and the child tears at its skin in a frenzy, drawing blood with its finger nails. This distressing sight and sleeplessness give rise to intense anxiety in the parents.

Climatic changes are of importance. Cold, frosty weather aggravates the eczema and more new patients are seen in the months February to April than at other times in the year. Intense heat also brings problems, possibly because in the inflamed, red, oedematous skin there is interference with sweating.

Prognosis of atopic eczema. Although many of the milder cases clear spontaneously by the age of two, the eruption in those who do not clear tends to leave the face but persists in the flexures and on the fingers. Persistent scratching, mostly at night, causes lichenification and the hall mark of atopic eczema is a leathery, pigmented but dry erythema in the flexures and around the neck. Although symptoms in most patients begin in childhood, a small group have no abnormality until after puberty. Clinical features in these patients do not differ from those who have started in infancy and the absence of a previous history should not preclude the diagnosis. The ultimate prognosis of atopic eczema is not too depressing. There is no definite time for it to remit and from the age of 2 onwards some clear each year. In a review of some 500 patients seen in childhood with infantile eczema, only 10 per cent had a significant disability 10 years later. Prognosis is un-favourable in those with a bad family history, where there are adverse psychological factors and in the group with a late onset of symptoms.

Not every eczematous eruption in an infant is infantile eczema and the following conditions may cause confusion:

(i) *Miliaria*. It is usual for infants between the ages of 4 to 6 weeks to develop groups of pinhead sized pustules around the nose and mouth, the so called milk spots. Occasionally this condition occurs over the whole body surface giving rise to erythema and multiple follicular pustules. The good general condition of the infant is in contrast to the alarming appearance of the pustular eruption. The condition is self-limiting and it subsides spontaneously without the use of antibiotics. The onset of the eruption on the face can simulate infantile eczema. The pustular lesions and the age of the infant should serve to differ-entiate the two conditions.

(ii) *Traumatic dermatitis*. Many children with a tendency to ichthyosis develop chapping easily in cold weather. This occurs on the exposed parts and red scaly eruption around the mouth and cheeks can simulate

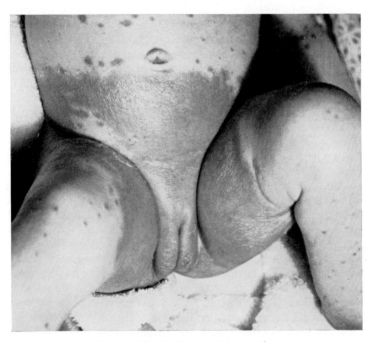

FIG. 28.—Psoriasiform napkin eruption.

infantile eczema. The absence of severe irritation and the speedy resolution with simple emollients should exclude the atopic state.

(iii) *Infective intertrigo* (or seborrhoeic eczema of infants). This condition resembles seborrhoea of adults in that the eruption starts on the scalp and spreads to the retroauricular folds, the creases of the neck, the axillae and the napkin area. The lesions are not vesicular but consist of raw, red exuding areas with crusting. Infection with bacteria and candida may be the precipitating cause, though it has been shown that the pH of the skin surface is more alkaline than usual and this being the underlying fault. The condition responds to combined antibiotic and corticosteroid applications and clears much earlier than infantile eczema.

(iv) *Psoriatic napkin eruption.* A dry, scaly psoriatic eruption appearing primarily on the napkin area but also involving the scalp, face and trunk has been noticed in recent years. The sites affected, the onset in the first weeks of life and the psoriatic appearance differentiate it from eczema. The recent increased incidence coincides with a rise of candida infections in infants and it is probable that this organism plays some part in the etiology. The condition clears spontaneously as the infant reaches the age of 4–5 months but applications of ung. Nystaform HC do hasten recovery. Powerful steroids should be avoided as they may cause skin atrophy. Despite the appearance there is little evidence that psoriasis will occur later in life.

Complications. Secondary infection of excoriated atopic eczema by pyogenic organisms commonly occurs and this often follows on a respiratory infection of virus origin and the exanthemata. Pyogenic infection can be recognised by pustule formation and the infection has an aggravating effect on the eczema itself.

Eczema vaccinatum

Of particular importance is the liability of atopic eczema subjects to develop severe and even fatal infections due to herpes simplex and vaccinia viruses. Though it is difficult to prevent accidental infection with herpes simplex, no patient with active eczema should be vaccinated against smallpox and contact between infants with eczema and recently vaccinated siblings and adults should be prevented. The viraemia produces fever and prostration accompanied by a pock-like eruption mainly, but not entirely, confined to the areas of the eczema.

TREATMENT OF ATOPIC ECZEMA

In no skin condition is the general management of the patient and the relatives more important than in infantile eczema. Over-anxiety and even a feeling of guilt that the child should be so afflicted is present in the parents of most atopic children. It is just as important to correct the parents' misconception about the disease and the handling of the child, as it is to apply soothing applications to the skin. Infantile eczema children have above average intelligence, they are over-active, aggressive, yet insecure and sensitive. Even without eczema they are difficult to handle and sleep less than normal children. At the first interview, time must be spent in explanation to the parents that this is an inherited defect which is not their fault and which has compensations in that the child may well be clever. The parents are also told that it is an error to over-protect the child, who should be encouraged to live a normal life. One of the most important points is correction of sleeping habits. Mothers often attempt to prevent their infants scratching by placing the cot beside their beds and holding the child's hands. This is the beginning of a bad habit; whenever possible, the baby should sleep in a separate room. In order to cut down nocturnal skin damage and to allow the family rest, mild sedation of the infant with an antihistamine elixir is necessary. Elixir of diphenhydramine hydrochloride (Benadryl) 10 mg. or elixir of promethazine hydrochloride (Phenergan), 5 mg. at night are suitable. These infants cannot easily be sedated by barbiturates, which should be avoided.

Diet. The great majority of children with infantile eczema can eat a normal diet and if the child is thriving, no change should be made. Very occasionally there is a history that one food, for example fish, produces swelling of the child's face. It is noteworthy that such food allergies produce an urticarial reaction and do not aggravate the eczema, but obviously this food should be avoided. Although positive reactions to scratch tests may be given to various foods, elimination of such a food from the diet does not improve the eczema and it is because of this experience that skin tests and elimination diets have largely been abandoned.

Local treatment. It is unusual today to see a baby with severely crusted eczema, but crusts, if present, can be removed by applications of equal parts of lead diachylon plaster and soft paraffin applied thickly on lint strips and left in position for 24 hours. The crusts adhere to the lint and any which remain on the skin are so softened that they can be cleaned off easily with gauze soaked in liquid paraffin. Once the crusts have been removed, the treatment of choice for the child's head and face is 1% hydrocortisone ointment. This should be applied sparingly 3 times a day at first and the intervals between treatments gradually lengthened. No ill effects have been seen after hydrocortisone has been applied for years and parents can be reassured about this. Standard strength fluocinolone acetonide (Synalar) and betamethasone valerate (Betnovate) applications may produce skin atrophy and adrenal suppression. They should be used only for short periods and once controlled the eczema may respond either to simple emollients or to

1 in 10 dilution of Synalar or Betnovate in a base such as cetomacrogol cream.

If obvious secondary infection is present, combined antibiotic corticosteroid ointment should be substituted, but if sepsis is very widespread, then systemic antibiotics are indicated. Whilst similar methods can be used on the limbs, it is often an advantage to occlude these with coal tar occlusive bandages covered with Tubegauze. If expertly applied, these may stay on for a week at a time. Such occlusive dressings have made unnecessary any other form of restraint and, above all, the child should not be tied to its cot.

There is considerable difference of opinion as to the effect of soap and water on babies with eczema. In winter weather and in ichthyotic infants soap should be avoided. Where there is a very bad history of eczema in the family, it may be advisable to clean the skin with emulsifying ointment or a proprietary cleansing cream. For general use, one of the less alkaline soaps is to be preferred. Even when the eczema is under control, the skin of many infants remains dry and cracks easily in cold weather. Oily cream B.P. or Boots E. 45 base are clean, easily applied emollients which can be rubbed in at bed time and before the child goes out into cold winds.

Parents often ask whether children with eczema can be immunised. It is safe to immunise against tetanus, diphtheria, whooping cough and poliomyelitis, but it must again be stressed that vaccination should not be carried out if there is any active eczema and it should be avoided, if possible, even later in life. Active immunisation to tetanus should be encouraged, because sufferers from atopic eczema react adversely to tetanus antitoxin.

Atopic eczema in older children and in adults is handled in the same way as in infants. There may however be psychological stresses which have an adverse effect on the eczema and these should be investigated. In the very severe cases where the disability interferes with all work and leisure activities, it may be justifiable to suppress the eczema by long term systemic corticosteroid treatment. This should never be used in childhood and, in our experience, has been quite unnecessary.

Napkin dermatitis

Though strictly out of place in this chapter, napkin rash may conveniently be dealt with adjacent to infantile eczema. Napkin rash is primarily a traumatic dermatitis due to friction and contact with material soaked in a highly alkaline solution. Frequent loose stools from over-feeding may irritate the skin and organisms in the faeces which split urea into ammonia increase the alkalinity. Soap which may be inadequately rinsed from the napkins is another source of alkali.

Sharply demarcated, dry, red and scaly patches on the lower abdomen,

48   SEBORRHOEIC ECZEMA

buttocks and convexity of the thighs is the usual clinical picture. The skin in the folds of the groin and the natal cleft which is unaffected, stands out strikingly. A less common type with punched out ulcers and vesicular, and even granulomatous papules, may cause difficulty in diagnosis, since it can raise the suspicion of syphilis or chicken-pox. A third variety, the psoriatic eruption has already been described (page 45).

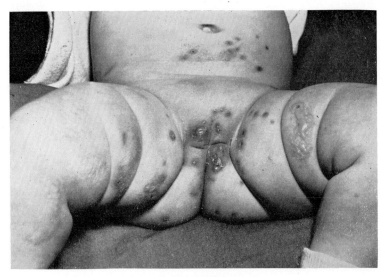

FIG. 29.—Bullous napkin eruption.

Treatment. In mild cases which occur very commonly, more care in rinsing the napkins and the application of a simple emollient, such as zinc and castor oil cream and correction of the over-feeding, is all that is necessary. Where there is infection, soaking the napkins in an antiseptic and the application of an antiseptic corticosteroid ointment, e.g. Vioform hydrocortisone, at each napkin change will succeed. The ulcerated and granulomatous type may not respond to these measures but will clear with painting of the napkin area with $\frac{1}{2}\%$ silver nitrate solution 3 times a day. As this method stains the napkins, it should be reserved for the rare case where other treatments have failed.

Seborrhoeic eczema
Despite its name the relationship of seborrhoeic eruptions and sebum flow is not yet clear, but it remains a useful descriptive term for

a clinical syndrome which is an inborn abnormality for which the mechanism remains a mystery.

The hormonal changes at puberty stimulate the sebaceous glands to enlarge and over-secrete and a temporary period of dandruff, greasiness of the skin and acne vulgaris is almost a normal phase of development. But in those with an exaggerated seborrhoeic tendency the sebaceous glands remain over-active and enlarged in the adult and the scalp is constantly covered with greasy scales. An important part of the syndrome is an increased liability to superficial pyogenic infection. Should any skin inflammation arise in individuals who have inherited the tendency, it will take on the pattern of a seborrhoeic eczema. Thus a

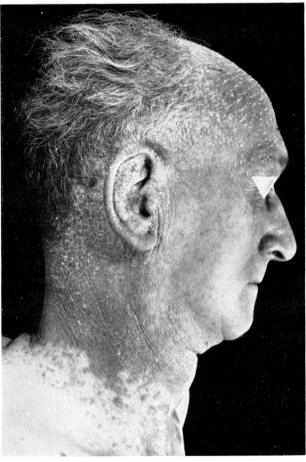

FIG. 30.—Seborrhoeic eczema.

dust dermatitis occurring in a seborrhoeic individual will resemble the seborrhoeic eruption.

Seborrhoeic eruptions are seen frequently after upper respiratory and pyogenic infections and in this way resemble acute guttate psoriasis. They are also adversely affected by anxiety states and mental depression. The relationship with psoriasis can be carried even further because there may be alternation of the two diseases in the same patient. The parts of the body affected by seborrhoeic eruptions are those which have the largest number of sebaceous glands, the scalp, the central part of the face, the sternal and interscapular areas of the trunk. Also often involved are the axillae and groins which are richly supplied with apocrine sweat glands.

The scalp is most constantly affected by a dry, white, scaly dandruff and for long periods this may be the only evidence of a seborrhoeic tendency. It may be difficult to distinguish this condition from psoriasis, though psoriasis of the scalp is usually patchy and the scaly lesions palpable. It is wise however to reconsider the diagnosis in any condition of dandruff which does not respond to the usual methods of treatment.

Another cause of scaling of the scalp is atopic eczema and ichthyosis which can produce an appearance very similar to that occurring in seborrhoeic conditions. A history of infantile eczema and evidence of flexural lesions on the rest of the body will help to distinguish between the two. An acute exudative eczema of the scalp, which resembles impetigo in its weeping of yellow seropurulent material which dries like lacquer on the hair, can arise in those who have seborrhoea of the scalp.

During the acute phase the eruption may extend to the face and ears, where confluent sheets of erythema and crusts involve the pinnae and external auditory canals.

The diagnosis can be confirmed by the finding of annular, greasy, scaly patches in the sternal area or follicular, erythematous papules on the chest and back. Often in association with an acute flare-up a generalised annular scaly eruption appears on the trunk, indistinguishable from pityriasis rosea. The stigmata of the chronic seborrhoeic state are all evidence of chronic pyogenic infection such as blepharitis, folliculitis of the beard, fissures at the nasolabial folds, the angles of the mouth and above and below the pinnae and chronic otitis externa.

Seborrhoeic intertrigo. Moist red intertrigo of the body clefts, the sub-mammary areas, the groins, umbilicus and axillae may occur in association with widespread seborrhoeic lesions or alone. When there is no evidence of seborrhoea elsewhere, it is difficult to differentiate it from flexural psoriasis or infection with candida or tinea and a mycological examination may be required.

TREATMENT

Numerous shampoos have been advocated for the control of dandruff but recurrences are the rule and most patients need repeated treatments every few days. The mild cases respond to twice weekly washing with 2% Cetrimide (Cetavlon) or similar detergent shampoos.

Selenium sulphide is successful in the control of dry scaling but is contra-indicated if active eczema is present. A spirit based hair lotion allays itching, but if the scalp is very scaly, a cream such as acid salicylic, and sulphur 2% of each in aqueous cream B.P. is more effective. This is clean water-soluble cream which can be used as a brilliantine.

Pyogenic infection plays such a large part in exacerbating seborrhoeic eczema of scalp and face that it is our custom to use Tetracycline

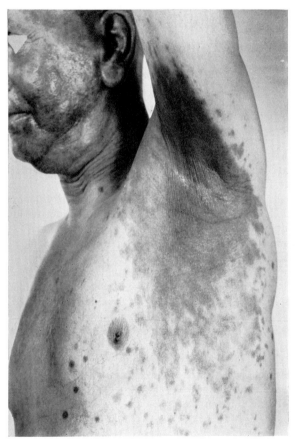

FIG. 31.—Seborrhoeic intertrigo.

hydrocortisone (Terracortril) ointment but other antibiotics such as gentamicin or sodium fusidate combined with a steroid may be equally suitable.

They can also be advised for lesions of the face. As a general principle, sulphur containing preparations are effective and calamine lotion with 2% sulphur can be used for lesions on the body.

The most pleasant treatment for intertrigo of the body folds is a steroid antiseptic ointment. Because so often candida is present as well as staphylococci one of those active against both organisms should be selected. Rarely in difficult cases recourse may be had to Magenta paint B.P. (Castellani's basic fuchsin paint).

There is a tradition that seborrhoeic eruptions can be alleviated by diet but this has not been our experience and unless the patient has diabetes or is grossly overweight, no dietetic restrictions are indicated. Far more important is the consideration of emotional factors. The seborrhoeic individual tends to be a depressive and treatment of the depression, if present, will benefit the skin condition.

Otitis externa

The lining of the external auditory meatus is skin and the auditory canal is affected by extension from adjacent regions of skin diseases such as seborrhoeic eczema or psoriasis, and occasionally by contact dermatitis from hearing aids, stethoscopes and medicaments. Fortunately, the purulent discharge from otitis media rarely causes otitis externa and the most common cause is trivial superficial bacterial infection. This leads to irritation and weeping, and the oedema of the meatal walls narrows the orifice and makes access for examination and treatment difficult. If furuncles complicate the infective dermatitis, severe pain and deafness occur.

Treatment. The principle of treatment is that of any infective eczema and today the most effective remedy is an antibiotic steroid ointment. We prefer ointment to drops and it should be gently wiped into the meatus after the canal has been mopped dry. If improvement is not rapid, bacteriological investigation should be carried out and meanwhile nystatin can be added to the ointment to control a possible secondary invasion by candida. It should always be kept in mind that dermatitis to a medicament or its ointment base may have developed. If this is suspected simple cleansing and the use of hydrocortisone 1% lotion only is often effective. Furunculosis of the meatus should be treated by systemic antibiotics, and any associated seborrhoea or psoriasis of the scalp and adjacent skin must also be treated.

CHAPTER 6

BACTERIAL INFECTIONS

THE skin is normally colonised by an innumerable flora of organisms most of which are harmless saprophytes such as anaerobic gram-positive cocci, diphtheroid bacilli, staphylococcus albus, candida and the acne bacillus. These reside in crypts, hair follicles, sebaceous glands and their ducts and their number and distribution varies with climate, age, hygiene, clothing and from one site to another. This resident flora is only temporarily reduced by scrubbing or the application of antiseptics.

In addition, there is a transient flora largely confined to more exposed areas and including potential pathogens such as haemolytic streptococci, staphylococci etc. The healthy human skin disinfects itself, destroying haemolytic streptococci with unsaturated fatty acids contained in sebum and staphylococci by desiccation so that this transient flora is only able to establish itself for a few hours and may be got rid of by washing with soap and water or more effectively by hexachlorophane. In a heavily contaminated environment such as a hosptal ward, transient pathogens may acquire temporary resident status. If the skin remains healthy such a state may be short lived, but if a breach of continuity of the skin occurs, or if the defence mechanism is impaired by a skin disease, active infection of the skin may take place.

Staphylococcal infection

Nasal carriage of pathogenic staphylococci is the most important source of infection. Over half the population are nasal carriers and contamination of their skin and especially their hands disseminates the organisms. Spread of infection is aided in winter by the sudden increase in upper respiratory infections and these have been found to coincide with increased skin sepsis.

Impetigo

The type of infection produced by staphylococci depends on the soil and the seed. In children impetigo is common, though it occasionally occurs in adults. About 80 per cent of cases are found to be due to staphylococci of phage type 71. A build-up of carriage of such a potentially infective strain in the nostrils of nursing staff or the umbilici of babies in a neonatal nursery may lead to an outbreak of impetigo among the babies, whose resistance to staphylococcal infection is negligible even though the skin of the new born is colonised by

53

non-pathogenic staphylococci within a few days of birth. Widespread blistered areas result which become denuded and crusted with serum. Blistering is such a feature of impetigo in this age group that it is called "pemphigus neonatorum". Certain strains of phage-type 71 staphylococci produce a delta toxin which in children can produce widespread erythroderma in areas unaffected by impetiginous crusting leading to fragility and shedding of sheets of epidermis (toxic epidermal necrolysis or Lyell-Ritter's disease).

In older children it seems possible that the initial lesion occurs in skin damaged by injury, or some other lesion such as herpes simplex. Once established the organism gains virulence by "passage" and is then capable of infecting the skin of susceptible contacts.

Uncomplicated impetigo usually appears on the exposed areas of face, hands and knees as delicate vesicles which rupture so rapidly that

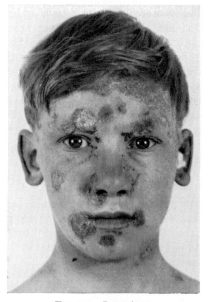

Fig. 32.—Impetigo.

they are rarely seen intact. Serous exudation coagulates in a honey coloured crust and the edge of the lesion may spread, still giving the appearance of a broken blister at the edge, with crusting proximal to this and healing at the centre of the lesion, which may thus produce circinate or gyrate patterns; during the active stage of the disease fresh lesions appear and spread daily. The skin beyond the lesions is normal unless secondary infection with haemolytic streptococci occurs, in which case crusting becomes more severe and an inflammatory halo appears round the lesions; in these cases there is also regional lymphadenitis.

In the adult in the tropics, heat and maceration of the skin cause such an increased activity of the disease that bullous lesions appear, which can become as widespread as those in the newborn.

Presence of skin damage from some other cause commonly provides an entry for the infection; atopic eczema becomes "impetiginised" producing a crusted mess in which the role of infection may be overlooked. The presence of pediculosis capitis may be missed even more easily and should be looked for in every case of impetigo of the scalp.

Secondary invasion of the lesions by streptococci of certain strains may give rise to acute glomerulonephritis. For this reason impetigo in neonates and in older children when the lesions look inflamed and extensive, should be treated with systemic penicillin. The staphylococcus is penicillin-resistant in a high proportion of cases, therefore local treatment with an antibiotic such as neomycin-bacitracin ointment should be applied 3 times daily after soaking off the crusts with liquid paraffin. If the crusts are thick equal parts of lead diachylon plaster and soft paraffin should be applied as a poultice spread thickly on strips of lint, moulded and bandaged on the affected area and left in place for 24 hours. The crusts are easily wiped off when it is removed. The lesions should heal in about 5 days but the child should be kept away from school until healed as this disease is contagious among children. In tropical climates even the infected adult may require systemic antibiotics to combat the staphylococcus.

Furunculosis

Boils are uncommon in small children and do not begin to be troublesome until the pilosebaceous apparatus becomes active at puberty. Once the skin has become colonised by pathogenic staphylococci, friction seems to be one of the precipitating causes and is most obvious in the "salt water boils" of deep sea fishermen; these occur in groups round the wrists where stiff wet oilskins rub the water-macerated skin. Even in those not exposed to such discomfort the wrist is a common site for boils, but the majority occur on the face, head and neck. In males 26 per cent of boils occur on the neck but only 4 per cent in females which suggests that friction of collars and trauma from the barber's clippers play an important initiating role. Nasal carriage of staphylococci occurs in the majority of those developing boils and is an important reservoir for auto-inoculation with organisms and for spread of organisms in a home or community.

Once a boil is established on the skin, the traditional methods of treatment would appear designed to spread infection, the application of kaolin poultices macerating and warming the surrounding skin, or occlusion under adhesive plaster producing a poultice of pus. It is therefore hardly surprising that one boil is often followed by many others.

Furunculosis may be a complication of some other disorders of which diabetes mellitus is the most important and the urine should always be tested to exclude this. Rarely furunculosis may be the presenting symptom of leukaemia, in which case the boils fail to resolve and become indolent ulcers with infiltrated edges, the infiltration being produced by invasion of the lesions with leukaemia cells. Such lesions may or may not be accompanied by enlarged lymph nodes or spleen, but should always be an indication for a blood count. Skin damaged by eczema or dermatitis is much more susceptible to invasion by staphylococci and furunculosis is a common complication of such cases. The skin disease may not be obvious and it should be remembered that hidden patches of eczema and lesions caused by pruritis ani or pruritis vulvae may be the nidus of infection.

Treatment should be aimed at preventing surface spread of infection and eradicating nasal carriage. It is desirable to have the antibiotic sensitivities of the staphylococcus estimated, especially if the patient has been in hospital recently, as the organism may be resistant to many of the broad spectrum antibiotics. If sensitive, the organism can be cleared from the anterior nares by the daily application of chlortetracycline ointment (Aureomycin). Chlortetracycline ointment should be applied to and about an inch around any boils or pimples until they have completely healed. Sticking plaster should be avoided as a dressing and if some cover is necessary gauze and bandage should be used. Hexachlorophane soap helps to reduce the carriage of pathogens and this substance may also be used as a dusting powder, and is available in sachets for addition to bath water. Such a regime usually brings recurrences of boils to an end in about 4 weeks in the majority of patients where there is no complicating factor.

Systemic antibiotic therapy has little effect in shortening the life of a boil and none at all in preventing recurrences, the only indications for systemic therapy being severe regional lymphadenopathy or progression of a boil to a carbuncle with surrounding cellulitis. Systemic penicillin therapy is usually adequate to deal with this since penicillin resistance is unusual in boils unless they have developed while the patient is in hospital. If penicillin is contra-indicated by resistance of the organism or sensitivity of the patient, tetracycline is the treatment of choice.

In patients with widespread eczema and boils any local steroid therapy should be combined with an antibiotic such as neomycin to prevent spread of sepsis. In these patients local antibiotic may not be sufficient to prevent spread of infection or the nature of the skin lesions may make such applications undesirable, in which case systemic antibiotics usually suppress infection and healing of the eczema prevents recurrence.

Infection of the apocrine glands in the axillae may occur in association with, or without, boils elsewhere. Tender red nodules are formed which may become large abscesses and cause great discomfort. Application of sodium fucidate ointment (Fucidin), painting with silver nitrate paint and systemic administration of tetracycline will usually heal these lesions, but if fluctuant the abscesses may require incision.

Finally, there remain those patients in whom foci of staphylococci have been dealt with and complications disproved, but who still continue to develop boils. These people seem to have an abnormally low resistance to staphylococcal infection which may be due to an immunological abnormality. Generalised ultraviolet-light therapy sometimes

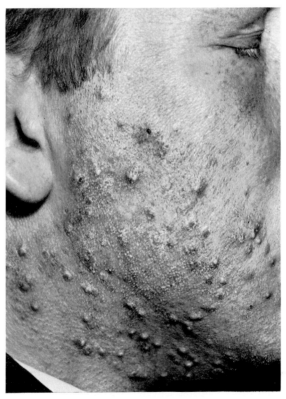

FIG. 33.—Sycosis barbae.

helps either by increasing their resistance or by sterilising the skin
The use of autogenous vaccines has been proved valueless in controlled
trials.

Sycosis barbae

This condition is now considerably less of a problem than it was
before the advent of antibiotics. It is a chronic staphylococcal infection
of the beard area, initiated by shaving and while this might appear
to make it an exclusively masculine disease it is occasionally seen in
women who shave. Chronic nasal infection and staphylococcal carriage
may be the precipitating cause, most obviously in those whose mous-
tache area is mainly affected. In many cases the disease is associated
with seborrhoeic dermatitis and there may be foci of sepsis on the skin
such as boils, blepharitis and otitis externa.

The lesions consist of small follicular pustules on a background of
erythema, the localisation to the beard area is marked and in long
standing cases some areas may become scarred and permanently epi-
lated. Scaling and crusting may also be present and hypertrophic
cellulitis and scarring may produce the fig-like appearance from which
the name is derived.

Eradication of sepsis elsewhere and the application of chlortetracycline ointment (Aureomycin) usually heal the lesions rapidly. In long
standing cases a residual erythema may persist which is controlled by
the addition of a local steroid to the antibiotic. The patient should be
encouraged to shave during treatment and an electric razor is preferable.
If the staphylococcus is tetracycline resistant a local antiseptic such as
iodochlorhydroxyquinoline ointment (Vioform) may have to be used.

Streptococcal infections

Streptococcal infection of the skin fluctuates from year to year in
accordance with the marked fluctuations in the incidence of other
streptococcal infections such as tonsillitis and scarlet fever. It is
most commonly seen as a secondary invader, causing inflammation
round the lesions of impetigo, or again in association with the staphylococcus, causing crusted ulcers scattered over the limbs known as
ecthyma.

Erysipelas can occur in any area of the body where a break in the
skin allows streptococci to gain entry but usually this break is a fissure
at the eye, ear, nostril or angle of the mouth. The patient becomes
acutely ill with high fever and rigors, sometimes before there is much
evidence of skin infection. From the fissure of entry an indurated
area of erythema, hot to the touch, spreads over the face, its spreading
border being easily palpable and the oedema of the dermis causing an
orange-skin appearance. Occasionally blisters may appear and in

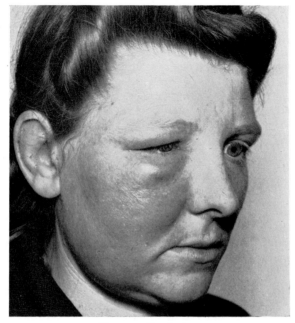

FIG. 34.—Erysipelas.

about 48 hours at least half the face may be involved, with oedema of the eyelids closing the eyes.

A course of systemic penicillin controls this dramatically.

Recurrent attacks, sub-acute in onset and with little constitutional disturbance may occur on the face giving rise to a less demarkated erythema. Treatment of the fissure of entry with chlortetracycline ointment (Aureomycin) until it is completely healed prevents recurrence, though some cases may require prolonged systemic therapy with sulphonamides. The systemic use of chlortetracycline is less reliable as about 40 per cent of haemolytic streptococci are now resistant to this antibiotic.

Long standing recurrences may damage lymphatic drainage of the face and produce chronic lymphatic oedema of the ears, eyelids or lips.

Recurrent cellulitis

Recurrent cellulitis, like recurrent erysipelas, is a streptococcal infection depending on some portal of entry in the skin. Most commonly it affects a leg, entering through fissuring between the toes usually due to tinea pedis. Like recurrent erysipelas, the infection may damage lymphatic drainage, each attack leaving increasing residual oedema which increases the likelihood of spread of infection in the next attack. Many of these patients can be shown to have a congenitally deficient lymphatic drainage.

The attacks are acute in onset with rigors and high fever which often precede the obvious signs of the disease; the inguinal lymph nodes become enlarged and painful, the foot and lower leg oedematous, red and slightly tender, the redness having a poorly defined border.

In the acute stage systemic penicillin therapy controls the infection, tinea pedis if present should be treated (q.v.) and the fissures healed. If chronic lymphatic oedema is established, massage and wearing of an elastic web bandage help to reduce this. In some cases prolonged systemic antibiotic therapy may be indicated.

Erysipeloid

Is an infection with a Gram positive rod *Erysipelothrix rhusiopathiae*, which enters through a cut or abrasion, usually on the hand. The infection is acquired from handling uncooked fish, shell fish, meat or poultry and is therefore encountered in fishermen, fishmongers, butchers and cooks. Starting at the site of abrasion a purplish red erythema with a well defined raised edge travels slowly over first one finger, then spreads to creep up other fingers and over the hand. The areas first affected tend to heal. There is usually no systemic disturbance which, with the slowness of spread, distinguishes this from erysipelas. The localised form lasts 2–4 weeks. Treatment with full doses of systemic penicillin overcomes the infection.

Tuberculosis

Tuberculosis of the skin was a major dermatological problem before the Second World War and is now a rarity.

Primary tuberculosis of the skin produces a small persistent sore at the site of inoculation, the indolent undermined edges of which are now more familiar in unhealed B.C.G. vaccination sites; the regional lymph nodes enlarge and suppurate. Most primary lesions are found on the lower limbs.

Lupus vulgaris most commonly develops in children between the ages of 2 and 15 years and it is probable that many cases are a secondary extension of a primary lesion though some result from blood borne spread of infection. The face and neck are the common sites but the lesion may appear anywhere. The affected area is red, telangiectatic and slightly scaly; when blood is expressed with a glass slide the small brownish (apple-jelly colour) nodules of individual tubercles can be seen. Scarring follows resolution in some areas and is an important feature. The skin forms an unfavourable environment for the tubercle

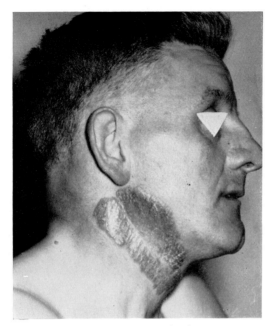

FIG. 35.—Lupus vulgaris.

bacillus, possibly because of exposure to light or low temperature and strains of tubercle bacilli isolated from skin lesions show an attenuated virulence. Progress of lupus vulgaris is therefore very slow and when it has arisen in childhood it is often accepted by the patient as a "birthmark".

Inoculation into the skin of adults who have already been sensitised or immunised by commoner primary pulmonary or alimentary infection produces warty plaques, whose bluish inflammatory halo is a clue to their possibly tuberculous origin. Once fairly commonly seen on the wrists of farmers and caused by contact with tuberculous cattle, lupus verrucosa cutis is now rare.

Treatment. All forms of tuberculosis of the skin respond to the administration of antituberculous drugs and, although the administration of isoniazid mg. 100 three times daily is effective, it is wiser to use a combination with P.A.S. If the lesion is ulcerated or there is evidence of active tuberculosis elsewhere streptomycin should also be given.

Syphilis

Syphilis in its early stages has become uncommon in Britain except in the larger ports, where infection is brought in from abroad and in the cities with shifting populations; nevertheless the possibility of sporadic outbreaks should be remembered.

The primary sore or chancre is nearly always acquired by sexual intercourse or kissing and appears after about 3 to 5 weeks at the site of infection. The sites usually affected are the penis or the vulva but 44 per cent of chancres in women are cervical and not easy to detect. Extragenital lesions occur on lips, fingers and anus, the latter being an increasingly common site as syphilis has become rife among homosexual males. The chancre is an erosion, ulcer or papule, rarely over 1 cm. in diameter, with an indurated base which can be lifted up like a button in the skin. About one week after its appearance one or more of the regional lymph nodes develops a rubbery painless enlargement.

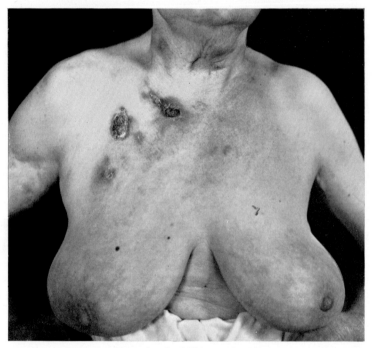

Fig. 36.—Syphilitic gummata.

Five to 6 weeks after the chancre, by which time this primary sore is healing, secondary manifestations appear as the result of dissemination of the organism throughout the blood stream. The rash may consist of macules, papules or scaly lesions but a mixture of these in a polymorphic eruption, lack of itching and a universal distribution are the characteristic points to be borne in mind.

The macular eruption appears at an early stage as pink or copper coloured, round or oval macules with an ill-defined edge, distributed on trunk, limbs, palms and soles. The lesions may be so delicate that they are difficult to see unless examined in daylight. Associated with the macules are papules or lenticular papules, these being a similar coppery or pink colour slightly scaly and characteristically infiltrated. In the later stages of secondary syphilis, numerous patterns of more florid papules and psoriasiform lesions may occur; the tendency to grouping and annular patterning of these lesions should arouse suspicions of the diagnosis. With the rash the patient often complains of vague malaise, headaches and pains in the limbs. There is generalised painless enlargement of lymph nodes, the epitrochlear glands being one of the characteristic groups enlarged. The buccal mucosa develops superficial erosions sometimes presenting as red patches and sometimes covered with mucous secretion which is likened to a snail track. Care should be taken to fold back the lips and examine their mucosal aspects. Condylomata lata are found in the perianal and vulval areas, but may occur at the angles of the mouth or in any of the flexures. They consist of flat moist plaques and nodules, often purplish in colour. In the later stages of secondary syphilis there may be a diffuse but patchy fall of hair, giving a moth-eaten appearance to the male scalp.

Late cutaneous manifestations of syphilis appear 2 to 10 years after the infection, the most common forming serpiginous or arcuate nodular lesions, which may be slightly scaly or ulcerated. In the central area over which they have passed they leave scarring and the lesion may be mistaken for lupus vulgaris especially if it occurs on the face or neck, but it traverses in months an area which would take lupus years. Gummata may be found in association with the nodular lesions or alone. Starting as a small nodule in the subcutis a gumma enlarges, becomes red and eventually ulcerates forming a discrete punched-out circinate ulcer with a slough at the base. A unilateral hyperkeratosis of palm or sole is a rare manifestation of tertiary syphilis. Leukoplakia predominantly affecting the tongue may also be a manifestation of the tertiary stage, though in these days other forms of chronic irritation such as trauma from dentures and smoking are a more common cause. The tongue is atrophic, sometimes scarred and sheets of white thickened epithelium involve the tongue and buccal mucosa. Whatever its cause this change in the mouth is potentially neoplastic. The most serious of all types of late syphilis is involvement of the cardiovascular and nervous system and although the skin can be the only organ involved, a careful examination of other systems must always be made.

Congenital syphilis is now seen very rarely owing to routine antenatal serological examination. The earliest cutaneous manifestation is a coppery coloured bullous eruption on the palms and soles appearing a few days after birth. The liver is usually enlarged and the child may have a serous nasal discharge, "snuffles", which obstructs breathing. A few weeks after birth the eruptions and other signs of secondary syphilis appear and changes in the long bones can be demonstrated on X-ray to consist of osteochondritis and periostitis.

The most rapid confirmation of the diagnosis of primary syphilis can be made by scarifying or abrading the sore and examining the serous discharge microscopically by dark ground illumination for spirochaetes.

In secondary syphilis the Wassermann and Kahn reactions are positive in virtually every case, spirochaetes can also be detected by expressing serum from condylomata. In tertiary syphilis the W.R. is positive in 90 per cent of cases and in cases of doubt the *Treponema pallidum* immobilisation test should be performed.

Because of the importance of tracing contacts the help of a specialist should be sought in treatment which is nowadays mainly dependent on penicillin in massive dosage.

Leprosy

With improved ease of travel and recent immigration from the Commonwealth, leprosy is increasingly encountered in Britain and though rare, its recognition is of obvious importance. It should be thought of in unusual skin eruptions in those from tropical or sub-tropical countries. Spread of the disease depends on the opportunity for contact with open cases of this infection and the greater the intimacy of contact the greater the chance of infection; spread of infection may also occur because of a high genetic susceptibility. Such conditions make the natives of these countries more prone to infection than transient visitors.

Fortunately the form of the disease most frequently seen in Great Britain is tuberculoid, occurring in patients with an adequate degree of resistance to the disease and a negligible chance of transmitting the infection. Sharply defined asymmetrical areas of hypopigmentation of the skin with a dry, slightly scaly surface; or infiltrated lesions with a sharply demarcated erythematous edge or forming a hypopigmented plaque are the common skin eruptions in this form of the disease. It is important to notice that while the macules resemble vitiligo, pigment has not completely disappeared. When such lesions are tested for sensation there is usually impairment of the senses of light touch, temperature and sometimes to pain induced by pin prick. In the presence of such skin lesions the ulnar, peroneal or great auricular nerves may be enlarged and easily palpable; if damage to these nerves is sufficient, foot drop or ulnar palsy may also be found.

At the other end of the scale is the patient with lepromatous leprosy in whom the tissue defences are overwhelmed by infection. Here the early skin lesions are symmetrical, small, vague edged, erythematous macules with a smooth and slightly shiny surface. Even at this stage there is a slight degree of infiltration which becomes more marked as the disease progresses to form plaques and nodules associated with diffuse infiltration of the facial tissues and pinnae. Polyneuritis is a late manifestation in this type of disease. Between these two extreme pictures is a spectrum of intermediate forms.

Diagnosis is established by biopsy of the skin, tuberculoid leprosy showing circumscribed dermal foci of epithelioid cells surrounded by histiocytes and lymphocytes in which bacilli are difficult to detect. Lepromatous leprosy shows a dense dermal infiltrate of vacuolated cells which distort and destroy epidermal appendages and are teeming with acid fast bacilli. In this stage nasal ulceration may occur and scrapings from the nose show profuse bacilli.

Because of the social implications of the disease, final diagnosis and treatment should be on the advice of an expert. Sulphone therapy is successful in the majority of cases and in recent years other drugs such as thiambutosine have proved effective.

CHAPTER 7

VIRUS INFECTIONS

Warts

Warts are the only human tumours which are undoubtedly due to a virus and like other tumours are due to uncontrolled proliferation of a race of altered cells. It has been known for decades that warts can be transmitted by cell-free filtrates and it is now possible to view the virus

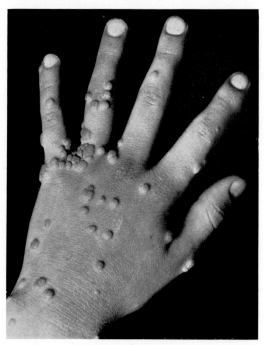

FIG. 37.—Warts.

particles by electron microscopy. The spread of warts in the school-age group has amounted to a plague in recent years and the incidence of lesions in the population is between 7 and 10 per cent or even higher in institutional groups. Spread of infection occurs in hand-holding school games, possibly through fomites and where warts on the feet are concerned, from walking barefoot on school gymnasium floors and swimming baths.

About two-thirds of any given crop of warts will resolve in 2 years, but in the same patient new warts may appear while others are resolving, so that it is more likely that spontaneous disappearance is due to an abiotic change in the virus than due to destruction of the virus by development of antibodies. On some hosts spontaneous disappearance may therefore be expected in 2 years, but others continue to develop fresh lesions for years.

Warts are commonest on the hand and their appearance there is too well known to need description. Occasionally paronychial warts may simulate an infective paronychia, but careful observation reveals the papilliferous part of the wart.

Plane warts are commonest on the backs of the hands and the face, appearing as flat topped, angular, smooth papules, either the colour of normal skin or light brown. Linear groups of papules are characteristic and caused by inoculation of the virus into scratches.

Vulval, perianal and penile warts proliferate into small cauliflower-like moist papillomata (condylomata acuminata).

Plantar warts occur mainly on the weight bearing area of the soles and may occur at the site of some minor trauma from a shoe nail. Owing to pressure they are unable to proliferate on the surface and so bury themselves into the sole, causing discomfort on walking. A plantar wart may be solitary and grow to a centimetre or more in diameter. Spread of lesions seems facilitated by hyperhidrosis and either small scattered seedlings may occur or a mosaic group of small warts may be formed.

Callosities often cause difficulty in differentiation but they are usually found on the transverse arch, nearly always symmetrically situated on both feet and associated with some minor foot deformity such as pes planus. On paring the surface of a callosity the keratin remains transparent and yellow, while the pared plantar wart reveals its papillae as minute bleeding points.

Treatment. As the majority of warts resolve spontaneously it is advisable in young children to play for time. Since any treatment, even a hospital out-patient appointment entails some form of suggestion, it is impossible to prove whether such white magic works, but the prescription of a simple ointment such as 10% salicylic acid in soft paraffin and the suggestion that the warts will have gone in a month is successful in about 30 per cent of children, particularly if the warts are plane.

Application of a CO_2 snow stick to the wart until a rim of frozen skin appears at its base will destroy those on the limbs, or a more successful method of freezing is with liquid nitrogen, a swab dipped in this and applied to the wart for 5–10 seconds producing a very effective reaction. Large warts on the fingers may need local anaesthetic infiltrated into the base and can then be scraped off with a curette, leaving a smooth bleeding base which should be cauterised with an electrocautery or silver nitrate stick.

The treatment of choice for plantar warts is soaking in 3% formalin. The solution is placed undiluted into an old tin lid or saucer, the scales

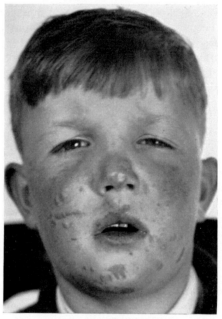

FIG. 38.—Plane warts.

scraped from the surface of the wart with scissors or nail file and the area of the sole affected soaked in the solution for 20 minutes each night. In 4–6 weeks the majority of warts are extruded and when the warts are small and multiple the treatment should be continued for even longer if necessary. If formalin is unsuccessful the foot should be soaked in warm water and the wart pared down each night, then the following paint applied: lactic acid 1 part, salicylic acid 1 part, collodion 3 parts. If after about a week the wart becomes very sore the treatment should be stopped for a few days then recommenced. Large solitary warts may be spooned out with a curette under local anaesthetic but it is preferable to give even these a trial with formalin as even if not successful in destroying the wart it cuts down the recurrence rate after curetting.

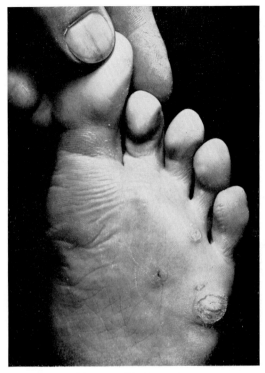

FIG. 39.—Plantar warts.

Filiform warts of the beard are sometimes very persistent and destruction with the diathermy or electrocautery at frequent intervals is indicated. Ano-genital warts should be painted with 25% podophyllin in spirit which is allowed to dry then thoroughly washed off with soap and water after 24 hours. The warts then rapidly resolve, though in a few cases with large long standing lesions, destruction by diathermy under general anaesthesia may be necessary.

Molluscum contagiosum

Molluscum contagiosum is caused by one of the largest viruses known to man. Transmission is commonest in swimming or Turkish baths and small, discrete pearly rounded nodules with umbilicated centres are produced, most commonly grouped in one area on the trunk. On squeezing the larger nodules a white curd-like substance is expressed consisting of degenerate epidermal cells containing many inclusion bodies. The lesions can be destroyed by freezing with liquid nitrogen

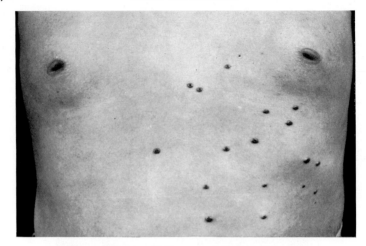

FIG. 40.—Molluscum contagiosum.

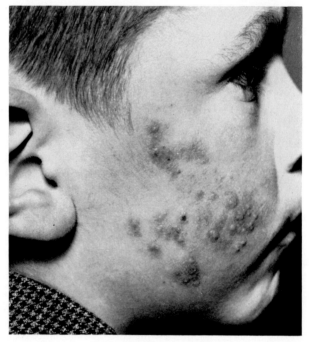

FIG. 41.—Herpes simplex.

or by spiking the umbilicated centres with a sharpened orange stick which has been dipped in pure phenol.

Herpes simplex

Herpes simplex is one of the commonest virus diseases of the skin and man is its natural host; over 60 per cent of people are infected and remain carriers throughout life.

Primary infection with the virus usually occurs in the first 5 years of life and may pass unnoticed. However, it can give rise to an acute gingivostomatitis associated with fever and local lymphadenitis. The lesions in the mouth resemble a profuse crop of small aphthous ulcers the gums are swollen and occasionally scanty vesicles may appear, dotted over the face and neck, uniform in size and leaving necrotic crusts after rupture. The primary lesion may involve the eye producing acute follicular conjunctivitis, which is usually self-limited.

The source of this infection can be traced in some cases to adult contacts who have suffered from recurrent herpes a few days before. In the early stages of this illness herpes antibody may be absent and a rising titre as the illness progresses is helpful in the diagnosis. Culture of the virus on chick embryo chorioallantois may also provide the answer in 3 or 4 days.

This primary infection subsides in about 10 to 14 days but the virus then remains latent in the epithelial cells of the buccal or nasal mucosa. In response to some stimulus these organisms may give rise to an attack of herpes simplex. Fever is the commonest stimulus but exposure to strong sunlight or emotional disturbance seems able to provoke an attack in some and it could be vasodilation rather than the temperature which is the uniting factor. The lesions appear at mucocutaneous junctions in many cases, but can occur in one area on the cheek, genitalia or even the trunk. A burning uncomfortable papule is succeeded by a group of small vesicles of uniform size which rapidly break leaving a crusted area, which usually heals in 7 to 10 days. When the secondary lesion involves the eye it may progress from conjunctivitis to keratitis and the formation of characteristic dendritic ulcers.

Those who suffer from recurrent herpes simplex have circulating herpes antibodies which show no rise in titre as the result of an attack of herpes simplex. In some cases erythema multiforme may follow about 10 days after the onset of the herpes (q.v.).

Treatment of the lesions is aimed at preventing secondary infection by using an antibiotic cream. There is no effective way of preventing recurrences though X-rays (to 300 rads) to the area of recurrence sometimes produce a long remission.

Eczema herpeticatum

The herpes simplex virus may also produce a secondary infection on skin damaged by eczema and is particularly prone to do so in babies. Contact in these cases has been with an adult suffering from herpes simplex, but vaccinia virus can produce an identical clinical picture if such infants are vaccinated or in contact with a person with a vaccination lesion. In the absence of guidance from the history only virus studies will distinguish the cause. The child with eczema becomes acutely ill with a high fever, the areas of eczema become vesicular and crusted and the local lymph nodes enlarged. The smallness, umbilication and uniformity of size of the vesicles and their tendency to group distinguishes this from pyogenic secondary infection. Fresh vesicles appear for as long as 9 days and are followed by necrotic crusts which are also similar in size.

Even the adult victim may be severely ill and in young babies this infection may be grave and death can occur from dehydration, secondary bacterial infection or adrenal necrosis.

This is the reason why infants with eczema should never be vaccinated against smallpox and should be protected from contact with anyone who has just been vaccinated. Similarly, sufferers from an attack of herpes simplex should be kept away from a case of infantile eczema or from any patient suffering from large, raw, weeping areas of dermatitis. There is no reason why the baby should not be inoculated against diphtheria, tetanus, whooping cough or poliomyelitis.

In eczema vaccinatum, smallpox gamma globulin administration ameliorates the condition and reduces the mortality and the thiosemicarbazones also appear to be of value in treatment. Both of these drugs may also be used prophyllactically if vaccination is essential in an eczema subject.

Herpes zoster

The virus causing herpes zoster is identical in size with that of chicken-pox and serological studies reveal no antigenic difference between the virus strains. It is therefore believed that zoster is due to activation of chicken-pox virus which has lain latent in the sensory ganglia since the primary infection years before. Zoster produces an earlier and greater antibody response because of the previous infection.

Chicken-pox is predominantly a disease of children between 2 and 6 years of age while herpes zoster is uncommon under the age of 15 years and more than half the cases are over 45 years old. Zoster may follow within 3 to 7 days of exposure to varicella, may follow damage to the dorsal nerve root by tuberculosis, tumour, leukaemia or arsenic or may appear for no obvious cause.

An attack is ushered in by pain over the nerve root distribution which usually lasts for about 3 days before the eruption appears; at this stage the regional lymph nodes are enlarged and tender. The rash follows a nerve distribution and may involve one or more derma-tomes, appearing in a continuous line or only in patches where the cutaneous nerves branch to the skin. Initially the eruption is a raised patch of erythema, but this is soon covered with a cluster of umbilicated vesicles which rapidly become purulent or haemorrhagic then form necrotic crusts. Pain usually continues with the eruption though some cases are remarkably free.

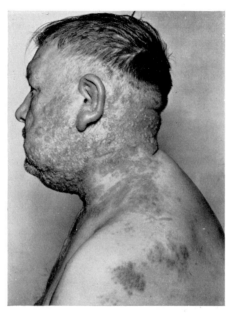

FIG. 42.—Herpes zoster.

On the thorax and abdomen this linear vesicular rash, stopping sharply at the midline back and front is easily diagnosed, but involve-ment of the trigeminal or cervical regions and the lumbosacral areas may be more puzzling.

The ophthalmic branch of the trigeminal nerve is that most commonly involved. Headache and tenderness of the scalp is followed by the characteristic eruption, usually in one sheet involving the forehead to the mid-line and extending back to the scalp. It is said that the eye is only involved if the nasociliary branch of the nerve is affected, pro-ducing vesicles down the side of the bridge of the nose. Involvement varies from trivial conjunctivitis to severe kerato-conjunctivitis or irido-cyclitis with secondary glaucoma. The eye is photophobic and irritable, with redness at the corneal margin. Patches of opacity may occur in the corneal substance and involvement of the iris is made apparent by sluggish reaction of the pupil or distortion of its margin.

Involvement of other ganglia may produce bizarre signs, the geni-culate ganglion being the least rarely affected, producing vesicles in the ear, external auditory canal and on the tongue, facial palsy and dis-turbances of hearing.

In patients whose resistance to infection is lowered, especially by reticulosis or leukaemia, the skin lesions may not remain localised but scattered discrete vesicles identical with those of chicken-pox may appear dotted over limbs and trunk. If this occurs as the presenting sign the patient should be investigated for possible underlying disease.

The skin lesions begin to resolve in about 10 days but healing may be slow in those cases where there has been severe necrosis and the resul-tant scarring may be especially disfiguring on the forehead.

Treatment in simple cases is aimed at preventing secondary sepsis by application of an antibiotic cream and relief of pain with Tabs. codeine co or Paracetamol. Pain and the discomfort of friction of clothes is diminished if the patient rests in bed.

If the lesions are mild and not secondarily infected the application of collodion or one of the modern occlusive dressing sprays diminishes the discomfort from friction of clothes, but such treatment can give rise to difficulties if infection occurs.

In herpes ophthalmicus the eye should be treated with 1% atropine sulphate drops twice daily and a local antibiotic eye ointment. If there is danger of ulceration of the cornea, specialist advice is required.

We do not advise the use of systemic corticosteroids in the treatment of this disease as there is no evidence that they shorten the duration of the skin lesions.

Neuralgic pain occasionally persists for months or years especially in the elderly. Analgesics are valueless in some cases and in these a form of counter irritation may be of value, freezing the affected seg-ment with ethyl chloride spray is the simplest of these methods. Such patients with post herpetic neuralgia suffer less when their minds are occupied and they should be encouraged to go about their normal daily tasks or be given some form of occupational therapy.

Orf

Orf is caused by the virus which produces contagious pustular dermatitis in sheep. Those infected are therefore usually sheep farmers, meat porters, butchers, or even occasionally housewives handling sheep's heads.

The lesions are usually single but can be multiple and are generally on the hand. The initial lesion is a dusky red papule which enlarges to 1 to 2 cm. in diameter and then resembles a large domed pustule. If the epidermis is incised the lesion is found to contain no pus but is solid with granulation tissue.

The disease is self limiting and resolves in 5 to 8 weeks. Treatment with compresses of $\frac{1}{2}\%$ silver nitrate lotion prevents secondary sepsis.

Complications of vaccination against smallpox

Mention has already been made of the development of eczema vaccinatum in atopic eczema subjects, but even the healthy occasionally suffer complications after vaccination. Generalised vaccinia is uncommon, developing in about 1:25,000; the eruption appears 9–14 days after vaccination and may crop for 2 or 3 days. The lesions may resemble variola but are usually more limited in extent. The prognosis is good and recovery usually takes place in the same time as the primary lesion but treatment with gamma globulin immediately stops further lesions. More commonly, an erythema multiforme or a morbilliform erythema develops 7–10 days after vaccination and fades rapidly. Accidental vaccinia may occur in incompletely immune contacts of the vaccinated person. The lesion goes through the same stages of a red irritable papule appearing four days later, becomes vesicular in 48 hours, increases in size and infiltration until it has become a pustule by the eighth to the eleventh day and then forms a necrotic crust. When such a lesion occurs on the face the inflammatory reaction and oedema are severe and the scar remaining may require plastic repair.

CHAPTER 8

FUNGUS INFECTIONS

THE fungi which can infect man are legion but we are concerned here with those common organisms which cause the various ringworm infections of the skin.

Candida albicans is normally a component of the flora of the human body, both cutaneous, oral, vaginal and intestinal and is in many cases transmitted to the child at birth. Alteration of the defense mechanisms by chronic diseases, immunological and hormonal abnormalities leads to the development of clinical forms of candidiasis.

Most of the ringworm fungi are transmitted from one person to another through direct or indirect contacts. Floors, duckboards, furniture, clothing, shoes and barbers' instruments contaminated with infected fragments of skin and hair are sources of infection for ringworm of the feet, body and scalp. Such transmission in a closed community like a boarding school can result in a rise in the rate of infection with ringworm of the feet from 5 to 36 per cent within 2 years. The importance of these sources of infection is also shown by the reduction in incidence among susceptibles when areas such as swimming bath floors are adequately cleaned.

Other infections are acquired from animals; cats and dogs being a source of the organism *microsporon canis* which causes ringworm of the scalp. Cattle, and in particular calves, are the source of *Trichophyton verrucosum*, causing cattle ringworm.

While the sources of infection are known, virtually nothing is known of the factors which determine the susceptibility or resistance of the host. In some cases superficial fungus infections recur year after year, while in others infection is brief; in addition, only a minority of those exposed become infected. Infection is followed by the development of hypersensitivity to the fungus and as this reaches its peak, in primary infections the lesion clears. Waning of immunity coincides with reduction in the degree of hypersensitivity but on reinfection the defences react quickly producing a rapid destruction of both host and fungus tissue and a rapid casting off of the infection. Whether resistance to infection is dependent on the sensitivity is not fully established.

Candidiasis (Moniliasis)

Candida infection may present in a variety of ways. In infants it is not uncommon in the first few weeks of life in the oral cavity, producing thrush in which milk white spots looking not unlike fungus cultures appear on the buccal mucosa and tongue; when scraped with a spatula these can be removed. In adults the same type of infection may follow antibiotic therapy, especially if oral and also may occur in patients taking corticosteroids. In both age groups nystatin oral suspension (100,000 units of nystatin per ml.) applied as a paint 4-hourly usually controls the infection rapidly.

In infants such an oral infection may be followed by the appearance of a flexural intertrigo, usually first attacking the groins and gluteal

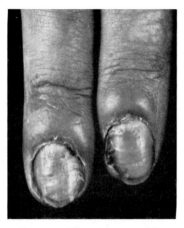

FIG. 43.—Chronic paronychia

cleft then axillae, folds of the chin and neck. Unlike a napkin eruption it is worse in the apex of the skin folds and forms a bright red glazed erythema with a demarkated but undermined edge. If severe, scattered scaly macules may appear on the trunk and scalp giving an ultimate appearance resembling psoriasis. *Candida* can usually be grown from the flexural lesions and treatment with nystatin cream or antiseptic steroid ointment thrice daily heals the lesions rapidly.

A similar intertrigo, often exuding serum, may be seen in the groins, natal cleft and sometimes spreading to the submammary areas and axillae in obese women. In such patients diabetes mellitus is usually the alteration in the soil which has allowed *Candida* to become a pathogen. It is important to observe the demarkated but slightly undermined edge to the lesion which looks as though it could have been vesicular. In severe cases psoriasiform macules may appear on the trunk as a sensitisation reaction and make the differential diagnosis from flexural psoriasis or seborrhoeic eczema difficult until the urine is tested. One sugar-free urinary specimen should not be accepted and if there is any doubt a glucose tolerance test should be performed.

The equivalent eruption is seen as balanitis in the uncircumcised male diabetic. *Candida* balanitis in the male also occurs in the absence of diabetes when exposed to chronic *Candida* infection of the vagina in his partner, which has been shown to be more prevalent in women on the contraceptive pill. The prolonged use of potent corticosteroid applications, particularly in the flexures, causes overgrowth of *candida* which often becomes the cause of chronicity of the lesion. Control of the diabetes is the most important measure and it is difficult to heal the eruption completely until this is achieved. Nystatin ointment is useful in mild cases and in more extensive lesions can be applied as a dusting powder. Where the lesion is very widespread 1% aqueous gentian violet can be applied as a paint but is a messy application.

The commonest area for *Candida* to cause trouble is the nail fold, producing chronic paronychia. Prolonged immersion of the hands in water frequently causes the quick to separate from the nail plate and the fungus becomes established in this area. Housewives, nurses, cooks, barmaids and bottle-washers are among those prone to develop this infection, the organism being acquired from the gastro-intestinal tract or sometimes associated with an active candida vaginitis. Once established, recurrent painful swelling appears at the base of the nail producing a red bolstered appearance; a bead of pus can be squeezed from this when active and damage to the nail bed causes the nail plate to become ridged and distorted. Rarely the organism may invade the nail plate causing it to become opaque, thickened and broken. Once one nail fold is affected others soon succumb until in severe cases all fingers are invaded.

Treatment is simply a matter of persuading the patient to keep the hands dry by using rubber or polythene gloves over cotton gloves for all wet work and to apply nystatin ointment or amphotericin B lotion to the nail folds at least 3 times daily so that there is constantly a film of medicament present. Other fungicides, such as Castellani's paint, can be used but are less acceptable because of their colour. The nail should not be removed except in those very rare cases where there is actual infection of the plate; the base should not be incised; poultices and hot soaks are the worst possible treatment as they increase wet and warmth.

In a number of cases the infection is a mixture of *Candida* and *Staph. pyogenes*. If the pain and swelling do not subside rapidly on treatment with nystatin, swabs should be taken for bacteriological examination and gentamycin ointment applied to the nail fold by day, nystatin ointment at night. If redness and pain are severe a course of oral erythromycin should also be given.

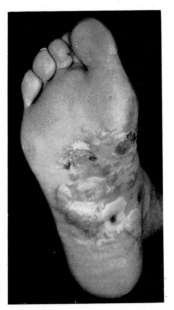

FIG. 44 (*a*).—Tinea pedis.

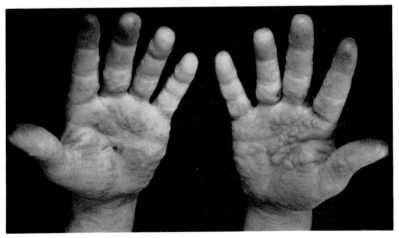

FIG. 44 (*b*).—Vesicular sensitisation of hands from tinea pedis.

Tinea pedis (Athlete's foot)

Tinea pedis is the commonest manifestation of fungus infection of the skin and occurs in those who bath communally regardless of athletic prowess. It is therefore common among boys at boarding schools, coal miners using pithead baths, workers using industrial shower baths as well as athletes in sports clubs. Three organisms are commonly the cause and all are mycelium forming; *Trichophyton mentagrophytes*, *Epidermophyton floccosum* and *Trichophyton rubrum*. Differentiation of the first two is unimportant as they produce a similar clinical picture and response to treatment, but *T. rubrum* can be considered separately on both accounts.

The earliest sign of tinea pedis is maceration scaling and sometimes fissuring on the webs of the little toes, usually worse on one foot. Such lesions may settle in cool weather and recur in the summer. Not all are due to mycelial fungi, as yeasts or even bacterial infection such as *Corynebacterium minutissimum* (erythrasma) may cause similar changes, microscopic examination revealing mycelium in only about 25 per cent of cases. Under adverse conditions such as warmth or prolonged immersion the infection may spread, usually first producing maceration between all the toes of the affected foot, then desquamation on the flexor aspect of the toes and finally clear loculated vesicles or even bullae on the instep. Both feet may be affected but asymmetry is characteristic.

At this stage secondary bacterial infection may also occur, the vesicles becoming purulent and the interdigital spaces exuding odoriferous serum. If this progresses further, cellulitis may produce hot, red swelling of the foot, lymphangitis and tender enlargement of the inguinal lymph nodes accompanied by pyrexia and constitutional disturbance. In the more severe stages of eruption sensitisation to the organism may give rise to a vesicular eruption on the sides of the fingers, later spreading to the palms (cheiropompholyx); if one foot is uninfected this will also become covered with vesicles on the soles and if the reaction is particularly severe a scaly macular eruption may appear mainly on the limbs, the individual lesions of which resemble pityriasis rosea.

Differential diagnosis. Although often treated with fungicides, not every eruption on the foot is tinea pedis; shoe dermatitis may produce chronic scaly or acute lesions with vesiculation and exudation. The important features which differentiate this from tinea pedis are its symmetry, the involvement of the dorsum of the toes rather than the webs and the pattern of the shoe on the sides of the feet. If the soles only are involved, as may occur from wearing rubber soled slippers, the weight bearing areas are affected and the instep spared, in converse to tinea pedis. Pustular psoriasis also gives rise to difficulties but this is also usually symmetrical, the pustules are uniform in size and evenly scattered over the red and scaly area of the sole involved; ringworm, by the nature of the activity of the fungus, being active at its edges.

Microscopic examination of the epidermis is desirable before treatment. The skin should be cleaned with methylated ether to remove debris and grease, then a scale taken from the active edge of the lesion or a vesicle snipped open and the roof removed to include the attached edge of the blister. Placed on a microscope slide, with the inside of the blister upwards, drops of 10% potassium hydroxide are added, the specimen covered with a coverslip and warmed slightly over a spirit lamp. Microscopic examination reveals branching threads of mycelium crossing the paving of epithelial cells, and if profuse forming a loose network.

Treatment depends on the severity of the attack and at its most severe the patient should be rested in bed as it is not possible to heal any acute eruption of the feet rapidly if the patient is up and about. In the acute vesicular stage the body is already making efforts to cast off the infection and too rapid destruction of the fungus with strong applications may exacerbate the sensitisation eruption. Wet dressings of sodium hypochlorite solution are sufficient at this stage and have the advantage of not staining the skin. If there is active cellulitis or bacterial secondary infection this may be combated with one of the broad spectrum antibiotics such as tetracycline. It is desirable to avoid penicillin in cases where a sensitisation eruption is established owing to its antigenic relationship to the sensitising trichophytin. The cheiropompholyx or macular sensitisation eruptions do not contain fungus and should be treated with thrice daily wet dressings of calamine or terra silica lotion.

As the acute infection subsides Castellani's paint should be applied to the feet and toes twice daily, the toes being kept separated by dry gauze. Once the stage of desquamation is reached the application of Whitfield's ointment twice daily removes the stain of the paint and any remaining traces of infection.

Where the reaction is less severe, but still vesicular, treatment should be started with Castellani's paint and in mild cases, where scaling of the toe webs is the only sign, Whitfield's ointment gives as good or better results than proprietary applications and is considerably cheaper. When the infection is slow to clear or keeps recurring, griseofulvin forte 500 mg. daily should be administered for at least 4 weeks.

Trichophyton rubrum infection

T. rubrum infection produces scaling between the toes but a more chronic, less reactive eruption on the soles, consisting of erythema and a dry scaling which characteristically confines itself to the

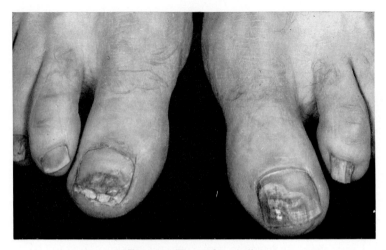

Fig. 45.—Tinea of toe-nails.

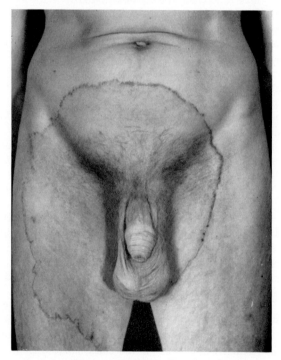

Fig. 46.—Tinea cruris, due to *T. rubrum* infection.

thickened keratin of the sole. In the majority of cases the nails are eventually involved producing opacity, yellow discoloration and subungual hyperkeratosis, starting at the distal end of the nail and progressing irregularly back down the nail plate. Eventually the plate becomes distorted and the condition spreads to involve other nails in an asymmetrical manner.

The hands usually eventually become involved, similar redness and scaling appearing on the palm and often remaining unilateral, the nail changes also produce a similar pattern. When both finger and toe nails are involved differentiation from psoriasis of the nails may be a problem, but in psoriasis the changes are usually symmetrical, pitting is a feature and finally, examination of cuttings from the nails in a potash preparation reveals whether fungus is present.

Extension of the *T. rubrum* infection to the legs produces a slightly scaly eruption dotted with follicular pustules, examination of a hair plucked from a pustule is more likely to reveal fungus than a skin scraping. When the groin is involved the condition spreads in an indolent fashion which may take months or even years to produce annular lesions extending often over the thighs and buttocks with a raised, slightly scaly edge. Locally applied fungicides have little effect on this organism and when this diagnosis is established Griseofulvin forte mg. 500 daily is the treatment of choice. Lesions of skin are usually controlled in about 4 to 6 weeks but nail plates need time to grow out, which may mean continuous treatment for 6 months before the finger nails become normal. Toe-nails rarely return to normal even after over a years treatment. If they are sufficiently distorted to be troublesome on this account removal of the nail under local anaesthesia followed by griseofulvin therapy until the nail has regrown is justifiable. Even prolonged medication with griseofulvin does not eradicate the organism from the toe webs and here all that can usefully be done is continuous application of Whitfield's ointment to keep it controlled.

Tinea cruris and Corporis

Spread of fungus infections to the limbs and trunk produces the annular or ringed lesions which led to their name. Tinea cruris (tinea of the groins) is much commoner in men and is usually caused by *T. mentagrophytes* spread from infections of the feet. Symmetrical red lesions with a raised scaly edge extend over each upper inner thigh. In warm climates this infection may spread to produce ringed lesions with a slightly vesicular edge on the trunk or limbs. In Britain such ringed lesions are usually derived from animal contact, the commonest being cattle ringworm and less commonly a *Microsporon canis* infection from kittens or puppies. Treatment of flexural and other eruptions with potent corticosteroid applications without establishing a definite diagnosis has greatly increased the incidence of widespread fungus infections in recent years, as the fungus thrives in such conditions.

Solitary lesions may respond to local fungicides but severe tinea cruris and widespread tinea circinata is an indication for griseofulvin in full doses, given for at least 6 weeks to prevent a recurrence.

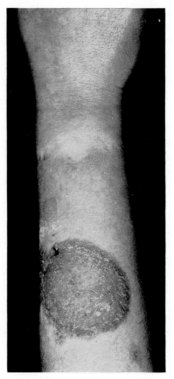

FIG. 47.—Ringworm.

Cattle ringworm is found not only in farmers who may have been in contact with infected calves but may be acquired from contact with farm gates, lorries used for conveying cattle, in the cattle market or abattoir. On the limbs it characteristically starts on the wrist, whence it spreads asymmetrically to the trunk, producing initially mild looking scaly rings which progress to heaped up pustule-dotted plaques. On the beard area the follicular reaction is more pronounced, producing round pustule dotted granuloma-like nodules and plaques; while in the scalp, especially in children, a boggy swelling known as a kerion is produced which may erroneously be incised as an abscess.

Such is the discomfort produced by these lesions and so slow is spontaneous recovery, taking in the case of tinea barbae up to 3 months, that griseofulvin therapy should be started at once. As a local application Castellani's paint is the most useful but sometimes secondary pyogenic infection may supervene and the appropriate local antibiotic may be required. Even with griseofulvin treatment lesions may last 4 to 5 weeks.

Ringworm of the scalp, of the types which were once commonly encountered, occurs only in children below the age of puberty and is cast off at puberty. It was becoming rare even before griseofulvin therapy was introduced and now that an effective, safe treatment is available it seems to have become even more uncommon. The usual infections are *Microsporon audouini*, derived from human vectors, or *M. canis* derived from cats, dogs or infected humans. An irregular bald area dotted with distorted broken stumps of hair appears, the degree of reaction in the underlying skin varying from very slight scaling in *Audouini* infections to erythema and scanty pustules in some *Canis* infections. Ringed lesions may also appear on the glabrous skin.

Examination of a hair stump in a potash preparation reveals it to be packed with spores. Examination under Wood's light (3300 to 3600 Å) produces a turquoise fluorescence of each infected hair. Such an examination is useful both in detecting fluorescent hairs for microscopy or culture and in detecting minor infections among contacts in a closed community such as a school or orphanage. If Wood's light is not available, or when one of the rarer types of ringworm of the scalp which does not cause fluorescence is suspected, it may be necessary to collect material for culture of the fungus. This can be done with a round polythene scalp massager which has been sterilised by immersion in 10% Teepol for 24 hours. The suspected scalp is massaged vigorously for a quarter of a minute. The polythene becomes electrostatically charged and picks up particles from the hair and scalp. The brush is then pressed into a dish of culture medium on which fungus cultures appear after incubation. *Canis* infections resolve spontaneously in about 3 months but before griseofulvin became available X-ray epilation was used for *Audouini* infections. Nowadays both infections respond to griseofulvin in the dose appropriate for the child's age and can usually be cleared in about a month.

Tinea versicolor

This is a trivial superficial infection with the organism *Malassezia furfur*. It is common in the tropics but also occurs in temperate climates. The lesions consist of faintly brown macules on the chest and back which may become confluent. The surface is very finely wrinkled. In pigmented skin partial depigmentation may occur. Examination with Wood's light imparts a yellowish green fluorescence to the lesions.

Scrapings mounted in potash reveal profuse short crescentic mycelium and clustered small round spores.

Treatment with half strength Whitfields ointment rapidly clears the lesions, but unless persisted in for several weeks they soon recur.

CHAPTER 9

INFESTATIONS

Scabies

Scabies is due to invasion of the epidermis by a mite *Acarus scabiei* (*Sarcoptes scabiei var. hominis*). The adult female is the form in which the mite is usually isolated and is approximately $\frac{1}{60}$ of an inch in length —just visible to the naked eye; the male is about half this size. Successful infection of a new victim is accomplished by a newly fertilized female which moves over the warm body at about 1 inch a minute until it selects a site for burrowing. This therefore requires fairly prolonged contact with an infected person and infection may be spread in hand holding games at school, as with a "venereal infection" and particularly between members of a family. Having burrowed into the horny layer of the skin the female remains in the burrow for the rest of her life. Two or 3 eggs a day are then layed for several weeks as the mite burrows along the skin. The eggs hatch in 3 to 4 days, the larvae then leaving the burrow and sheltering in hair follicles. The nymphs moult to give rise to the adult form. Mating occurs on the surface of the skin and the cycle recommences, the whole cycle from egg to oviparous female taking 14 days.

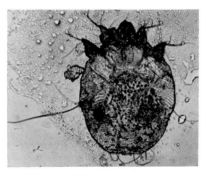

Fig. 48.—The acarus of scabies.

The mites burrow in certain parts of the body, the majority being found on the hands and wrists. The burrows are most visible on the sides of the fingers or the flexor aspect of the wrists. The other area in which burrows are most commonly found is the sole of the foot; they may also be found on elbows, buttocks and axillae. On the penis and scrotum the burrow is obliterated in an inflammatory nodule and such lesions in an itchy patient are virtually diagnostic. Similar nodules resembling small abscesses also appear scattered over the trunk in infants. In these areas there are very few acari and the average number on a sufferer is about 12; as 60 per cent of these are to be found on hands and wrists this is obviously the area to search first for burrows.

When the mite first burrows into the skin of a patient who has never before had scabies the infestation remains symptomless for about a month. After this an erythematous reaction occurs round the burrows, a papular urticarial eruption appears on the forearms, axillary folds, waist, inner thighs, buttocks and round the ankles. The patient

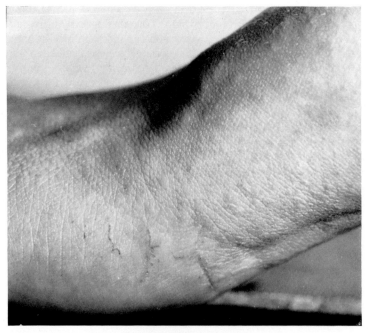

FIG. 49.—Scabies burrows.

then commences to itch, the irritation being most severe when warm in bed at night. This stage appears to be one of sensitisation of the host and in the presensitisation phase the host acts as a symptomless carrier. When such a sensitised patient acquires scabies on another occasion he develops a reaction within a few hours to the entry of the mite and may therefore scratch it out before further infestation can occur, thus developing a type of immunity by sensitisation.

The degree of reaction which follows sensitisation varies and when severe can cause vesiculation on the hands and feet, especially in children and a scratched eruption which may sometimes become eczematous on the limbs and trunk. If secondary pyogenic infection occurs, pustules and boils appear on the affected areas and it is not uncommon to see large ecthymatous ulcers on the buttocks.

In adults the rash is confined to trunk and limbs but in young babies lesions may appear on the face and scalp.

The distribution of the rash, the intense itching and the usual story of other affected members of the family should suggest the diagnosis, which can then be confirmed by isolating an acarus. A watchmaker's lens for magnification leaves both hands free; a good light and an ordinary pin are necessary. A search should be made on hands, wrists and feet until a burrow is found. At the anterior end of the burrow the mite is visible as a white oval with a black dot at its front. The burrow in this area is opened with the pin point and the acarus can easily be induced to adhere to the pin. Placed on a slide, a ring of ink round it makes it easier to find under the microscope, where it is not only satisfying evidence of a correct diagnosis but also a horrifying inducement to the patient to carry out treatment with meticulous care.

In mental defectives and psychotics infestation with the acarus becomes overwhelming, possibly because of a diminished sense of itching and therefore little scratching. In these patients the epidermis becomes thickened, crusted and infected and can be seen to be teeming with mites on biopsy even though actual burrows may be obliterated by infection and hard to find. Such cases may be diagnosed as eczema or even exfoliative dermatitis until they become recognised as the source of scabetic infection in others.

Treatment. Before carrying out treatment the nature of the infection should be explained to the patient and the importance of all in the household being treated whether yet itching or not.

On the first day a bath should be taken and the hands, wrists and feet scrubbed with a soft nail brush to open up burrows. After drying the skin benzyl benzoate lotion is applied to the whole body from the neck down, preferably with a paint brush by someone else, care being taken to cover every inch especially round hands and feet. This is allowed to dry and the same clothes then reworn.

On the second day the same procedure. On the third day, after bathing and painting, clean clothes should be worn and the dirty clothes washed or sent to the cleaners. Clean bedclothes should also be used and if the dirty blankets are not washed, storing them for a fortnight will ensure that any remaining acari are dead.

Stoving clothes is not necessary and it is probable that the impregnation with benzyl benzoate which the dirty clothes receive is sufficient to kill any wandering acari. Nevertheless, such a routine impresses upon the patient the need for care in treatment.

Itching should cease within a week and no more benzyl benzoate should be used, though if the itching subsides slowly calamine lotion with 1% phenol may be used to allay this. In babies and young children benzyl benzoate lotion applications sting unbearably and, when the family includes these, monosulfiram lotion (Tetmosol) should be used in the same routine as benzyl benzoate on all members of the family.

Scabies varies in its incidence over the years and, although most common during wars, its fluctuations are probably independent of national calamity (though some maintain that they presage calamity). From 1935 until the outbreak of war, scabies was already on the increase and wartime conditions determined its further spread. After the war it died out, until by 1950 it had become almost a rare disease. Ten years later it had again become much more common. It is possible that such fluctuations depend on the lowered incidence of sensitised individuals and the increase in non-immune carriers, institutions of various types acting as reservoirs of infection.

Pediculosis capitis

The head louse, although indistinguishable from the body louse localises to the scalp and its incidence is still remarkably high among school children in industrial areas where 15 to 20 per cent may be infested in the poorer areas of towns. The present vogue for lacquered piled hair, which may be undisturbed for weeks, is spreading this infestation among an older age group. Often infestation is symptomless, the clue being the presence of nits on the hair shafts. They are seen best with a magnifying glass as shiny, pearl-coloured, oval bodies with a cuff which embraces the hair shaft. In mild infestations the adult louse may not be found, but in more severe cases itching is intolerable, the scalp becomes secondarily infected, dotted with impetiginous crusts or even oozing over the whole scalp. The lymph nodes in the posterior triangles of the neck become enlarged and tender and usually in such cases the lice can be seen in the scalp. Sometimes a papular urticarial eruption may be present on the upper trunk or, more misleadingly, this may be a macular erythematous rash.

Treatment. The scalp should be washed each night for three successive nights in gamma benzene hexachloride (Lorexane shampoo). Each day after this the nits must be combed out using a Durbac comb until they are entirely removed. In cases where the scalp is secondarily infected an antibiotic cream is applied to the scalp when the hair has been dried after shampoo. It is rarely necessary to cut the hair, the cream can be applied to the scalp by parting the hair on one side, smearing cream down the parting, repeating the parting nearer the crown and continuing in this fashion until the whole scalp is covered.

Pediculosis corporis

Body lice are rarely seen in this country except in vagrants and unwashed eccentrics. The patient complains of generalised itching and the trunk and limbs are covered with excoriations and, in longstanding cases, pigmented. The lice arc more likely to be found in the clothes than on the body and the best way to make the diagnosis is to search the seams of the clothes where collections of the small pearly eggs are to be found.

Treatment. The patient should be bathed and calamine lotion with 1% phenol applied to relieve the itching. The clothing should be dusted with D.D.T. powder to prevent spread of the lice, then placed in a bag and sent for disinfestation by washing or stoving.

Pediculosis pubis

The crab louse affects the pubic hair causing intense itching in the genital area. It may also spread to other body hairs. In adults it spreads as a venereal infection.

Treatment. The affected areas should be washed for three successive days in gamma benzene hexachloride (Lorexane shampoo).

Papular urticaria

Many children after infancy and before puberty suffer attacks of papular urticaria. The lesions are small, round, shotty wheals which may blister, commonly called 'heat spots', often ascribed to food allergies, they are in fact what they look like—multiple insect bites. A careful search will usually show lines of lesions along which the insect has fed.

Reactions to insect bites vary according to the degree of sensitivity of the sufferer. Infants are not sensitised and show little reaction; the sensitised adult produces an itchy urticarial lump within half-an-hour of being bitten. Between these two stages is one of delayed hypersensitivity in which the reaction to a bite is delayed 48 hours and then produces a persistent urticarial papule which may not only last for many days but may be followed by a flare of activity in other previous insect bites. For this reason the lesions may be profuse.

Diagnosis. Allergic urticaria is unusual in childhood and its transient wheals which fade without trace are unlike the crusted papules of papular urticaria. When more than one child in a household is affected the condition may be confused with scabies but it is uncommon to see papular urticaria round the hands and wrists, whereas a careful

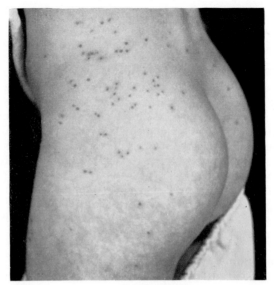

FIG. 50.—Papular urticaria.

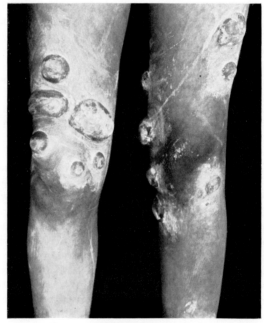

FIG. 51.—Bullous papular urticaria.

search in these areas will eventually reveal a scabies burrow from which an acarus can be prized. On the lower limbs large bullae may occur especially in girls. Other bullous diseases are uncommon in children and the only other bullous lesion likely to be seen is erythema multiforme which predominantly affects the upper limbs.

Just as demonstration of the acarus in scabies puts the diagnosis beyond argument so does demonstration of fleas from the domestic dog or cat allay the resentment with which the diagnosis of insect bites is often received. The parents should be instructed to brush the dog or cat over a sheet of black polythene and bring the brushings and hairs for inspection, when a search with a magnifying glass or microscope will usually be rewarding.

Treatment. Removal of the source of insects is the only cure. If this is the family dog or cat it should be dusted with an insecticide and any chairs or rugs on which it may have sat should be similarly dusted and vacuum cleaned. In the autumn midges in the garden, in the summer sand fleas at the seaside, mites from the family budgerigar, mites from birds' nests in the eaves of the house are all possible sources which must be eliminated. Where these are outside sources and uncontrollable the child can be protected with an insect repellant cream containing dimethylphthallate when it goes out to play. For crusting lesions antihistamines are of little value and the antipruritic effect of 1% phenol in calamine lotion is useful.

CHAPTER 10

URTICARIA AND PURPURA

Urticaria

Urticaria or nettlerash is characterised by an eruption of transient wheals and though frequently caused by hypersensitivity it is not always of allergic origin.

Wheals are formed by extreme dilatation of skin capillaries which allows serum to escape into the surrounding dermis. The dilatation is produced by histamine released from the mast cells of the dermis. An urticarial wheal can be artificially produced by the intradermal injection of a small quantity of histamine, and the release of tissue histamine may be provoked by a wide range of substances called histamine liberators, some of which are used therapeutically to cause counter irritation over arthritic joints. The capacity to release histamine is possessed by the alkaloids morphine and atropine and by many substances present in plants and animals.

Nettle stings, jelly fish stings and many insect bites cause local urticarial wheals by direct histamine liberation. It is believed that where an allergic mechanism is responsible, histamine is formed after the antigen–antibody reaction has taken place.

Allergic urticaria

The mechanism of urticaria differs from that of contact dermatitis in the following ways:

	Dermatitis	*Urticaria*
Route by which allergen reaches the tissue.	Surface contact.	Via the blood stream having been injected, ingested or inhaled.
Antibodies in serum.	Absent.	Present IgE or IgG.
Confirmatory test.	Patch test.	Scratch test or passive transfer test.
Time of response.	Delayed 48 hours.	Immediate.

It is always easier to understand a subject if a concrete example is taken and serum sickness illustrates the urticarial process well. Serum sickness is caused by the formation of antibodies to horse serum. After a latent period of 7–9 days, the time taken for sensitivity to develop, an acute generalised urticaria occurs, often the first lesion being on the site of the serum injection. Associated with the urticaria are fever, joint pains and occasionally lymphadenopathy and enlargement of the spleen. Antibodies to the serum can be demonstrated in vitro and sensitivity can be transferred by injecting some of the patient's serum into the skin of a non-sensitive person. If horse serum is then injected into the same site, an urticarial wheal reaction will occur immediately. This is known as the passive transfer test or the Prausnitz-Kustner reaction. A similar mechanism is responsible for acute urticaria which follows the consumption of unusual foods, e.g. strawberries, lobster and shellfish. Drugs are an even more common cause,

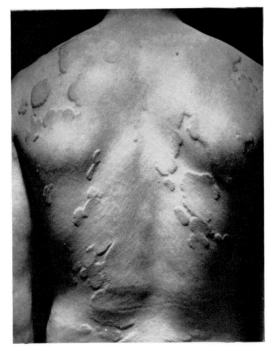

FIG. 52.—Urticaria.

penicillin being the most frequent offender at present and it is not generally realised that the time interval between the dose of penicillin and the onset of urticaria may be as long as 4 weeks.

Aspirin and salicylates have the capacity for potentiating any cause of urticaria. Thus, sudden recurrence in a well controlled case of urticaria may be due to aspirin unwittingly taken in a preparation such as Alka-Seltzer.

Urticaria may also occur as a reaction to the patient's own cellular products and this is seen after deep X-ray therapy to a neoplasm and

sometimes after severe bruising. A similar mechanism may be responsible for urticaria after acute infections such as tonsillitis, appendicitis
and associated with pregnancy and menstruation. Allergy to other
animal products occurs in parasitic disease such as hydatid and intestinal worm infestations.

Acute urticaria. Intense irritation ushers in the eruption of
wheals which may occur anywhere on the body surface. Wheals vary
in size from 2–3 mm. to several cm. across. Diagnosis may be difficult

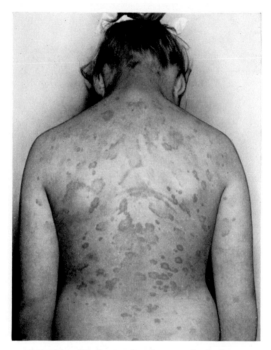

FIG. 53.—Urticaria, showing annular lesions.

if they tend to form rings. Wheals last 8–24 hours and fade without
trace, except in the most active urticaria where, on dependent parts of
the body, purpuric staining may occur. Joint swellings, fever and even
a palpable spleen and superficial lymph glands can accompany the
rash to give a clinical picture which resembles acute rheumatism or
glandular fever.

Differential diagnosis. The wheal is such a characteristic sign
that diagnosis should be simple. Ringed urticarial wheals may resemble
erythema multiforme but the history of transient lesions rather than

fixed ones should support the diagnosis of urticaria. Urticarial reactions confined to the shoulders and back should stimulate a search for lice on the scalp or on the underclothes and occasionally scabies can present as urticaria.

TYPES OF URTICARIA

Dermographia. An intensely severe triple response on scratching the skin so that whealing follows 5 minutes after a light scratch or friction with a towel. Often a lifelong condition it may follow acute urticaria and may be aggravated by emotional tension.

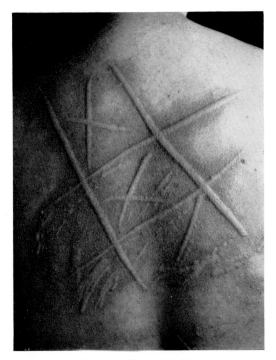

FIG. 54.—Dermographia.

Giant urticaria (Angioneurotic oedema). The urticarial lesions which may involve the subcutaneous tissues and swellings of the eyelids, lips, tongue and larynx occur without irritation or generalised urticaria. The dividing line between this condition and severe acute urticaria is a fine one. Some patients with giant urticaria have a family history of the complaint and in them nervous factors play an important role.

Heat and emotion (cholinergic) urticaria is a generalised eruption of small erythematous wheals precipitated by physical exercise, rise in body temperature or emotional tension. This is a disorder of the sympathetic control of sweat glands in which acetylcholine causes the liberation of histamine.

Solar and cold urticaria is an acquired hypersensitivity to actinic light or to cold and manifests itself as urticaria on exposure to sunlight or after bathing in cold water. When heat or cold is the precipitating factor the diagnosis can be confirmed by heating the patient under an electric blanket or immersing a limb in iced water. These conditions are particularly resistant to treatment.

Chronic urticaria. Many patients suffer from recurrent and prolonged attacks of urticaria throughout their lives. Some belong to the eczema, hay fever, asthma group but in others no such genetic weakness can be found. Whilst it is possible that occasionally an allergic cause such as penicillin in milk, or aspirin may be overlooked, thorough investigation, including elimination diets and the search for focal sepsis fails to elicit a cause in 80 per cent of such patients. Emotional factors are responsible in some and the possibility of family tension should be considered in the etiology.

Treatment. First find the cause. In a first attack this may be impossible but in successive attacks a case which incriminates a particular food or drug may be built up. Skin tests are valueless in this investigation but a good diary may be helpful. As has been mentioned above, in chronic urticaria, emotional stress may be the precipitating factor and steps must be taken to ease this if possible. Antihistamine drugs which block the cell receptors for histamine are of value in both acute and chronic urticaria but there are a large number of antihistamine drugs and it would be wise to learn to use one or two. In theory it should be possible to block the action of histamine in every patient, but undesirable side effects prevent very high dosage and in practice success is attained in about 80 per cent. Promethazine hydrochloride (Phenergan) has the advantage of long action and a sedative effect and it need be given only at night in a dose of 25 to 75 mg. When it is desirable for the patient to keep awake, chlorpheniramine maleate 4 mg. (Piriton) 6-hourly, cyproheptadine hydrochloride (Periactin) 4 mg. or triprolidine hydrochloride (Actidil) 2·5 mg. 4 times daily can all be used. In children antihistamines may be given in the form of elixirs rather than tablets. Once the urticaria has been controlled the dosage of antihistamine should be maintained for several days then slowly lowered. In chronic urticaria suppression by antihistamines may be needed for months or years but no untoward effects have been reported. In psychogenic urticaria, sedatives may be of more value than the anti-histamine drugs.

In very acute urticaria where there may be swelling of the tongue and glottis and peripheral vascular collapse adrenalin 0·5–1 ml. of a $\frac{1}{1000}$ solution injected subcutaneously is the treatment of choice and repeated every 2 hours. The use of systemic steroids in the treatment of urticaria is, we believe, unnecessary except in acute allergic crises which may occur in serum sickness and penicillin urticaria. In these circumstances, intravenous hydrocortisone is indicated. Local applications are of little value in the relief of symptoms but a tepid bath may give comfort.

Purpura

Purpura, like urticaria, is a physical sign and not a disease entity. It indicates the escape of red blood cells through the endothelial walls of dermal capillaries and the most important factor in all forms of purpura is the capillary wall. As long as this remains undamaged platelets can be removed or the blood made incoagulable without resultant purpura, but capillary endothelial cells and platelets are antigenically similar and are often damaged in the same pathological process. For the maintenance of normal capillary permeability vitamin C and calcium ions are necessary. A general increase of capillary weakness can be demonstrated by the Hess test in which a sphygmomanometer cuff is left on the arm for 5 minutes at a pressure of 80 mm. Hg, more than 10 petechiae below the cuff show an abnormal fragility.

Any intense dilatation of the capillaries will permit localised purpura and thus it is seen as a complication of urticaria, insect bites and cellulitis, and in many skin eruptions on the legs where the capillary pressure is high.

In most examples of generalised purpura more than one mechanism is at fault and any classification is of necessity arbitrary and incomplete. The following is based on the main pathogenic mechanisms.

1. *Congenital defects of capillary wall*
   Ehlers-Danlos Syndrome. A disorder of elastic tissue in which the skin is easily stretched and the extent of joint movements is abnormally large.
2. *Increased vascular permeability*
   Scurvy.
3. *Increased vascular fragility*
   Senile purpura.
   Corticosteroid purpura.
   Vascular purpura due to infections, drugs and systemic disease such as uraemia and diabetes.
   Textile purpura and itching purpura.

4. *Chronic vascular purpura*

Gravitational purpura. See page (148).

A number of little understood syndromes with eponymous titles such as Schamberg's Disease.

5. *Purpura due to autoimmune damage to vessel walls*

Henoch Schoenlein purpura. See page (116).

Allergic vasculitis.

This includes a number of syndromes in which the clinical signs are dependent upon the size of the vessels affected. Purpura is associated with urticarial papules, erythema and nodules which may ulcerate.

6. *Purpura due to quantitative deficiency of platelets*

This may be idiopathic or secondary to bone marrow depression by drugs, infections, radiation or bone marrow disease such as leukaemia.

7. *Purpura due to dysproteinaemias*

Disturbances of the plasma proteins may present with purpura mainly affecting the legs and often precipitated by exposure to cold.

8. *Purpura due to coagulation disorders.*

Acute purpura associated with fever and malaise is a medical emergency and the possibility of septicaemia or meningococcal meningitis should be the first consideration. These are rare conditions and the more probable cause of fever and vascular purpura is drug sensitivity. This may occur with or without thrombocytopenia.

Purpura as part of an auto-immune disorder can usually be distinguished by the occurrence of a variety of skin lesions. The earliest in most types of vasculitis are urticarial papules which only become purpuric after some hours. In the majority the Hess test is negative.

Thrombocytopenic purpura whether primary or secondary is likely to present with epistaxis or haemorrhages elsewhere in addition to the purpuric eruption which may be very extensive. The Hess test is usually positive.

Investigations in any case of purpura must include complete blood platelet and bone marrow examinations and estimations of serum proteins and immunoglobulins.

Many of the patients with purpura due to vascular fragility will give no positive findings in the laboratory and, even in those of drug origin, confirmation of the diagnosis is often impossible. Because of their clinical importance the following are worthy of mention.

Senile purpura. Prolonged exposure to sunlight weakens the collagen which supports the superficial dermal blood vessels. In the elderly spontaneous subcutaneous haemorrhages of varying size appear on the backs of the hands and the forearms. The haemorrhages are painless but cause anxiety because of their appearance. In association with senile purpura linear or star-shaped pseudo scars are often seen. Changes in the collagen similar to senile skin are produced by prolonged systemic or topical corticosteroid therapy.

Scurvy. The possibility of scurvy should be considered in any old person living alone and the first symptoms of scurvy are often mental depression and pain and swelling in the legs and ankles. The classical follicular haemorrhages may not be apparent but large ecchymoses, bruises and a curious tender woody feel of the muscles are found.

Purpuric dermatitis or itching purpura. A chronic eruption of papules, scales and purpuric haemorrhages, is seen quite frequently on the lower limbs. This eruption may occur spontaneously but it can also be produced as a contact reaction to clothing, possibly by some chemical used in the finish of cloth. It is also a very recognisable pattern of the drug eruption due to carbromal which, unlike most drug eruptions, persists for many weeks after the drug has been discontinued.

CHAPTER 11

DRUG ERUPTIONS

IN the past two decades more potent drugs have been produced than ever before and have brought with them their train of iatrogenic disease in every branch of medicine and surgery. Drug eruptions have now taken the place of syphilis as "the great mimic". In dealing with this problem two obvious facts should not be overlooked, the first being the history of having taken a drug and the second the maxim that any drug can cause any eruption.

An accurate history must be obtained from the patient of any medicament being taken whether orally, by injection, inunction or pessary. The word drug conjures up visions of opium and hashish to the laity therefore specific questions must be asked, especially about those more common drugs of addiction, aspirin and aperients. The dates on which any drug was commenced and stopped are of vital importance and the fact that a drug was stopped an interval before the onset of the eruption does not rule this out as the cause; penicillin may produce a reaction 2 or 3 weeks after injection, gold and organic arsenic can cause trouble weeks later.

Given the story of taking some drug its apparent harmlessness should not lead to its dismissal as a cause, for virtually every drug in the pharmacopoea has caused an eruption in someone.

The types of eruption produced are widely varied even when caused by the same drug, but when acute in onset certain features suggest the aetiology. Primarily the eruption is an allergic dermal reaction which may vary in its intensity from a widespread morbilliform erythema to an urticarial, purpuric or bullous reaction. Drugs, however, often produce a mixture of these reactions which is unlike any other skin disease and even the colour, which is often peculiarly vivid and purplish, suggests the diagnosis to the tutored eye.

While it is possible for a drug eruption to produce severe constitutional disturbance, this is not common and often the patient, covered with an alarming looking rash, suffering a drug fever with temperature well above 39°C, is sitting up in bed looking fit and well. Such an event during what was the convalescent period of another illness should lead to consideration of cessation of therapy, though unfortunately it may have the reverse effect. In a severe reaction generalised lymphadenopathy may occur and can lead to further confusion in diagnosis. In mild reactions to a drug which is rapidly excreted, the fever abates within about 24 hours of cessation of therapy and may be a better guide to the offending agent than the rash. This is especially useful in patients having polytherapy when it is undesirable to stop all the drugs at once.

It is impossible to list all the described reactions to commonly used drugs, but it is useful to consider the reactions in groups and have some idea of those more likely to be incriminated in each group.

The commonest reaction is a non-specific erythematous or morbilliform eruption and barbiturate drugs are the most widely used cause. The rash fades rapidly as soon as the drug is stopped in the majority of cases, but where there is impaired liver or kidney function especially in the elderly the outlook is not so good and will be discussed below.

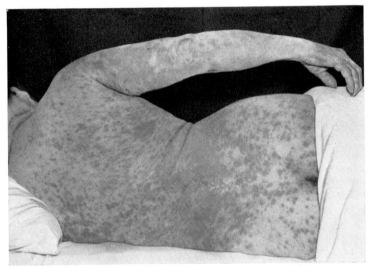

FIG. 55.—Maculo-papular drug eruption due to phenobarbitone.

Phenobarbitone sometimes produces a characteristic confluent erythema of the palms, soles and flexures in addition to the widespread morbilliform eruption. Sulphonamides commonly produce a similar eruption and so, less frequently, do some of the non-barbiturate hypnotics such as chloral and glutethimide (Doriden).

The next degree of severity is urticaria and in these days penicillin is the commonest drug to cause this. The illness which it produces is comparable with serum sickness, antitetanus serum being a cause which should diminish with its decreasing use. There is an interval of 10 days to 3 weeks or even more after the injection of penicillin, then an acute onset of urticaria, fever and severe flitting joint pains due to hydrarthrosis. If the patient has previously suffered urticaria caused by penicillin, the reaction may be almost immediate, starting with a wheal at the site of injection and followed in hours by a generalised eruption. Penicillin can provide the clearest example of the difference between epidermal and dermal sensitivity; if the patient has previously developed contact dermatitis due to application of penicillin to the skin, urticaria may accompany but behave independently of a resurrection of dermatitis in the previously affected area. Once this urticarial reaction is triggered off it may last for months or even years in those who have a predisposition to allergy as evidenced by other allergic responses such as asthma or hay fever or a family history of such diseases. In a few cases this prolongation may be due to further exposure to penicillin, milk being one possible source when the milk from penicillin treated cows is allowed into the normal supply. Ampicillin reactions have a similarly delayed onset but provoke a coppery maculopapular eruption, looking rather like severe pityriasis rosea. There is a particularly high incidence of this eruption when the drug is given in the course of glandular fever.

Aspirin is another common cause of urticaria though the incidence in relation to the amount consumed must be very low. Aspirin also acts as a histamine release agent and aggravates urticaria initiated by other causes so that sufferers from this eruption must be warned against the drug.

Bulla formation is largely a matter of degree of reaction and any rash, when sufficiently severe, can pour out enough serum to produce vesicles and bullae. However, some drugs seem to progress to this degree more frequently and here again sulphonamides and barbiturates are the common offenders. Often the eruption is a mixture of papules, urticaria and vesiculation; vesicle formation often starting on the hands and feet.

It is possible for drug-induced purpura to be caused by thrombocytopenia or by damage to capillary walls; in practice capillary damage as part of the dermal reaction is by far the commonest cause and therefore some degree of purpura is common in many severe drug eruptions and is partly responsible for their purplish colour. Phenylbutazone (Butazolidin) is very prone to produce a purpuric element and, on occasions, may produce a pure purpura. Several of the oral diuretics of the chlorothiazide group produce a purely purpuric and ecchymotic eruption and since they are often used in the presence of oedema of the legs the ecchymoses usually become necrotic and ulcerate.

One can now go on to more specific types of eruption in which it is possible to name the most likely cause. A fixed drug eruption is so called because on each exposure to the drug lesions recur on the same site. Usually they are raised discs of erythema which in a severe reaction may produce a solitary bulla at the centre. They arise within an hour or two of taking the drug and usually subside quickly when it is stopped, leaving a disc of pigmentation which may last until the next attack. On the skin the lesions may be solitary or scattered fairly profusely, they may also affect the mucosae, causing raw red patches on the buccal mucosa or urethritis. Phenolphthalein is the commonest cause being present in many purgatives, especially the "chocolate laxatives" and agar compounds. More obscurely it may be present as colouring matter in toothpaste and icing sugar. Phenacetin, phenazone, barbiturates, sulphonamides and tetracyclines may give rise to a similar eruption. Fixed drug eruptions are unusual in that a patch test of the offending agent applied to the area of the eruption will produce a reaction without any preparatory abrasion or stripping of the epidermis.

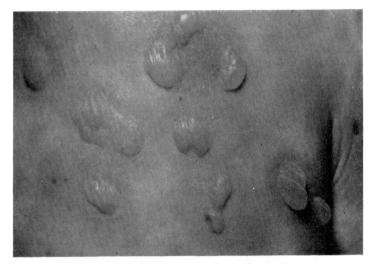

Fig. 56.—Bullous drug eruption—phenacetin.

Acneform papules and pustules especially on the face are produced by the halogens, particularly bromides also by the tuberculostatic drugs isoniazid and ethionamide. Iodides can also produce these lesions and are liable to aggravate an existing acne vulgaris, so that in cases where there has been a recent severe flare of acne it is worth enquiring whether "blood mixtures" or cough medicines which could contain iodides have been taken. Bromides also give rise to granulomatous plaques dotted with pustules on the shins known as bromoderma. Chronic poisoning with iodides will occur in all if the dose is high enough and given for long enough, but individual susceptibility varies and "iodism" may develop on a small dose giving rise to lachrymation, nasal catarrh and gastro-intestinal disturbance. Accompanying these symptoms granulomatous nodules may appear on the cheeks or in the nose. Halogens contained in modern drugs such as bromide salts of pentamethonium and probanthine and iodides in radio-opaque materials can produce these reactions.

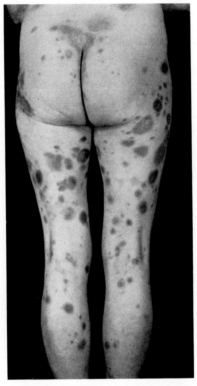

FIG. 57.—Drug eruption due to phenolphthalein.

Carbromal gives rise to a purpuric eruption in which there is also an epidermal involvement, causing faint erythema and scaling. An identical purpuric dermatitis can be produced by sensitivity to fabrics and was frequently caused by khaki during the Second World War; also a gravitational purpura may cause widespread capillary fragility and purpura on areas remote from the gravitational lesions on the lower limbs. In all three eruptions Hess' test of capillary fragility is positive. Differentiation depends on the distribution of the eruption and the history of taking Carbromal. Sedormid is now little used but produced not only a capillary fragility but also platelet clumping and thrombo-cytopenia which resulted in a similar purpuric eruption.

Lichen planus is described elsewhere in this book and the lichenoid eruption produced by drugs can be identical in appearance even to the mouth lesions. Gold salts and organic arsenic produce such an eruption which may last for months or years until the drug has been eliminated. Mepacrine and chloroquine also produce this eruption, the former staining the skin yellow which gives a clue to the drug but also being more slowly excreted the eruption lasts for months while that due to chloroquine usually resolves in a few weeks. Amiphenazole (Daptazole) and para-aminosalicyclic acid (P.A.S.) also give rise to a lichenoid eruption which fades rapidly after the drug is stopped. In the case of mepacrine and chloroquine itching of the skin and complaints of nausea or dyspepsia commonly precede the rash and should be taken as a warning to stop the drug.

Chronic poisoning with inorganic arsenic is rarely used as a therapy today but we are still seeing the late results of the use of arsenic in the treatment of psoriasis, dermatitis herpetiformis, "anaemia" and its addition to the epileptic's bromide mixture to prevent bromoderma. Such medication in the 1920's and 1930's now presents its results as a slate-grey speckled pigmentation of the skin, "raindrop pigmentation" as the subject is said to look as though rain has partly washed off engrimed dirt, hyperkeratoses of the palms and soles, multiple epithe-liomata—usually basal celled but sometimes intraepidermal squamous cell carcinomata and in some cases cirrhosis of the liver. There is also evidence to suggest that visceral carcinomata be more frequent in such patients. A slate-grey pigmentation of the light exposed areas of the skin also occurs after prolonged administration of chlorpromazine.

Generalised exfoliative dermatitis may be produced by any drug if its administration is continued after the skin has started to react, but in general it is the slowly excreted drug which gives rise to this degree of severe reaction. Gold and arsenic are the commonest offenders and in both early signs of toxic reaction should be watched for and the drug stopped if these occur; soreness of the tongue, angular stomatitis and the presence of albuminuria often precedes any skin eruption. The rash may start as an innocent looking morbilliform eruption which rapidly produces a confluent erythema affecting every inch of the skin, marked oedema of the subcutaneous tissues and generalised lympha-denopathy.

Mercury contained in teething powders was the cause of a syndrome known as Pink disease or acrodynia which occurred in children up to the age of 3 years. Irritability, photophobia, loss of hair and a tender swelling of the hands and feet with shiny erythema of these areas produced a characteristic picture which has disappeared since the inclusion of mercury was forbidden in these powders. Sporadic cases still occur from absorption of mercury in ointments.

Drug induced light sensitivity has been known since the sulphona-mide drugs produced it and nowadays the hypoglycaemic sulphona-mides used in the treatment of diabetes cause similar reactions, but the range of sensitisers is now much wider and includes chlorpromazine and all the antibiotics given systemically including penicillin and nalidixic acid; of these the highest incidence of light sensitisation has been observed with demethylchlortetracycline. The patient develops an eruption on the light exposed areas of face, neck and hands which may vary from a few papules to an acute erythema resembling severe sunburn. In some cases the eruption subsides when not exposed to strong light, but in most, once established the rash persists until the cause is withdrawn.

Other reactions which may be drug induced can also be toxic reactions to infective and other factors, these include erythema multiforme, erythema nodosum, polyarteritis nodosa and lupus erythematosus-like phenomena. These will all be discussed in the next chapter.

TREATMENT OF DRUG ERUPTIONS

Once the diagnosis has been established the majority of mild drug eruptions subside rapidly when the drug is stopped. Confirmation of the diagnosis by patch testing is only possible in a few examples such as fixed drug eruptions or after scarifying or stripping the epidermis in the case of sulphonamides. Intradermal injections of penicillin are not an accurate assessment of sensitivity and even in infinitesimal doses this procedure is fraught with dangers of inducing a severe reaction or anaphylactoid shock. Test doses of the suspected drug are similarly dangerous and only warrantable in such mild recurrent reactions as fixed drug eruptions in which the degree of sensitivity seems to be low. In general there are sufficient unrelated drugs available as alternative medication in these days to allow one to accept that the patient is sensitive without exposing him to the risk of additional proof.

Urticarial eruptions may be severe, particularly when induced by serum or penicillin. The patient should be rested in bed and given doses of antihistamines sufficient to bring the condition under control. In the presence of severe urticaria tolerance to these drugs seems to be raised and in an adult with a severe reaction a start can be made with cyproheptadine hydrochloride (Periactin) 8 mg. (2 tablets) three times daily and promethazine hydrochloride (Phenergan) 50 mg. (2 tablets) to night. Discomfort may be relieved by the application of calamine lation with 1% phenol and the dose of tablets reduced gradually once the urticaria is fully controlled. In some cases antihistamines fail to control the eruption in which case prednisolone should be given, starting with 30 mg. daily and reducing by one tablet each day once the eruption is controlled, at the same time adding or maintaining antihistamine therapy. It may be necessary for the sufferer from penicillin urticaria to continue on a small maintenance dose of antihistamine for weeks or months to prevent recurrence. Smaller doses of antihistamines may relieve the itching in other types of drug eruptions but do little to alter the course and duration.

Other widespread eruptions should be an indication for bed rest and if acute a blood count should be performed as drugs such as thiouracil may depress bone marrow function when the eruption produced is very mild. In the elderly or in the presence of poor liver or kidney function or sometimes because administration of the drug has not been stopped sufficiently early in the reaction, the eruption spreads rapidly and produces widespread severe erythema, ulceration of the mucosae, prostration and vasomotor collapse. The blood pressure may fall to a dangerously low level, unnoticed unless it is regularly checked, and if this happens, combined with the toxic effect of the drug it may produce kidney damage as severe as tubular necrosis. In severe drug eruptions such a course can usually be prevented by giving corticosteroid therapy without delay. A start should be made with prednisolone 30 to 40 mg. daily; if there is vomiting or diarrhoea it is better to give hydrocortisone intravenously. A careful watch must be maintained on fluid balance and serum electrolytes as well as the blood pressure.

Desensitisation is a dangerous and often unsuccessful process where dermal reactions are concerned and fortunately it is nearly always unnecessary. Epidermal reactions due to drugs such as penicillin can be of vital importance to doctors and nurses who are unable to avoid such contact and remain in their work. In such cases daily subcutaneous injection of penicillin soluble starting with 10 units per ml. and doubling the dose daily can be used to prevent further attacks of dermatitis.

Sensitivity to the offending drug is lifelong and it is important to impress upon the patient the need to warn any doctor prescribing for him of the allergy. Failure to do so may result not only in a recurrence of the skin eruption but in anaphylactic shock and possible sudden death.

CHAPTER 12

SKIN REACTIONS TO INFECTION AND INTERNAL DISEASE

THE skin has a range of pattern reactions which usually remain true to type but may be mixed; they are provoked by every conceivable toxin including drugs, systemic bacterial and virus infections, reticuloses, malignant neoplastic disease and as part of auto-immune reactions. The margins of definition are blurred, yet it is useful to define the separate reactions, as the commoner cause varies in each and the prognosis varies accordingly.

Erythema multiforme

This eruption is acute in onset, the extent of the lesions varies greatly, but the sites usually affected are the face, the flexor aspect of the forearms, hands in either aspect and knees. In very severe eruptions the whole body may be involved. As the name implies the lesions are

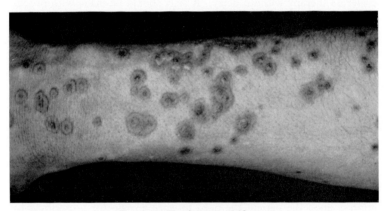

FIG. 58.—Erythema multiforme.

polymorphic; pink papules and slightly raised discs usually form some of the elements. The characteristic lesions are described as erythema iris and consist of annular red lesions with a purple centre which in time develops a play of colours similar to a bruise. When severe the centre of this target lesion consists of a vesicle or rarely a sizable bulla so that this is one of the causes of a blistering eruption.

The other characteristic of this reaction is involvement of the mucosae, usually the mouth only. The buccal mucosa is shed leaving a raw red surface to which shreds of mucosa still adhere; the tongue and red margin of the lips may be similarly affected, the lips rapidly becoming crusted by serous exudate. Similar changes can occur in the vulva and there may be urethritis. Involvement of the eyes may cause conjunctivitis, which can be sufficiently severe to produce adhesion between palpebral and bulbar conjunctivae; alternatively when precipitated by virus infection phlyctenular conjunctivitis can occur. Mucosal involvement of this type can occur in all three sites with no or very little involvement of the skin but is more common in severe reactions with a profuse eruption, pyrexia and profound constitutional disturbance. Various synonyms, including Stevens-Johnson syndrome, have been given to this wide range of reactions but they are better thought of as one entity.

Whether the attack is mild or severe it lasts for about 10 days, at the end of which time the lesions subside rapidly, though repair of the buccal mucosa is slower.

The commonest cause is a virus infection and in one-third of cases this is herpes simplex. There is an interval of about 10 days between the attack of herpes and the eruption of erythema multiforme, so that if mild the herpes may be forgotten unless a special enquiry is made, or if severe the mouth lesions of the toxic eruption may obscure the remains of the herpes. Herpes simplex being commonly recurrent the accompanying erythema multiforme may recur in greater or lesser degree with each attack though usually after a year or two the tendency to produce this toxic eruption subsides, even though the herpes continues to recur. Less commonly other virus infections such as virus pneumonia may precipitate this reaction and occasionally it may be seen in the prodromal stage of the exanthemata. *Str. haemolyticus* is an occasional cause, usually as finger pulp infection rather than tonsillitis, and *Mycoplasma pneumoniae* has been recovered from blister fluid in a small number of cases.

Drugs, in particular barbiturates and sulphonamides, are almost as common a cause as herpes simplex, giving rise to the complete clinical picture with mucosal involvement and they are the commonest cause of very severe attacks with constitutional disturbance. Some of the widespread fixed drug eruptions bear a close resemblance to erythema multiforme and in tracing the drug it must be remembered how prone to forget are the habitual patent medicine addicts. Toxic epidermal necrolysis (Lyell's syndrome) resembles severe erythema multiforme but is even more calamitous. The illness is preceded by fever and toxaemia, the whole body surface becomes a dusky red and the skin wrinkles and peels off in large sheets leaving a raw surface like a scald. In adults the majority of cases are drug-induced, phenylbutazone being the most commonly identified agent and 25 per cent of such cases die.

Other rare systemic diseases such as leukaemia and disseminated lupus erythematosus may give rise to erythema multiforme, so that if the cause is not obvious the patient should be investigated with such entities in mind.

TREATMENT

Those cases due to virus infection are often mild and the only treatment necessary is rest for a few days to enable an antipruritic lotion such as calamine lotion with 1% phenol to be applied. If itching is troublesome, antihistamines may relieve this but will do nothing to shorten the course of the disease.

Severe attacks are often the result of drug sensitivity which must be recognised and its administration stopped; but once triggered off this seems to be an "all or none" reaction and does not begin to improve until it has run its course of about 10 days.

Systemic steroid therapy has little or no effect in shortening the attack but is indicated if there is severe constitutional disturbance with pyrexia and signs of collapse with lowered blood pressure. In such a case prednisolone 30 mg. should be given each day until the condition is controlled, then gradually diminished and stopped. An antipruritic lotion is sufficient application except in those patients with large bullae. If tense, these should be pricked to allow the serum out in order to retain the roof as a cover for the erosion and an antibiotic cream applied to prevent secondary sepsis.

Mouth lesions are always uncomfortable and may necessitate a semi-fluid diet. The application of chlortetracycline 250 mg. in 10 ml. of water as a paint gives some relief.

Erythema nodosum

The onset of erythema nodosum is usually sudden and in all except the mildest attacks the patient is pyrexial and suffers flitting joint pains and sometimes joint swellings which are often erroneously supposed to be rheumatic. The lesions characteristically appear on the shins as red nodules, about the size of a penny. They are initially bright red and shining, but with the passage of time they may assume the same play of colours as a bruise and fade leaving bruise marks behind. Painful and throbbing when erupting they are very tender to touch. Oedema of the legs rapidly accompanies the nodules and can be severe if the patient persists in remaining ambulant. Usually the nodules are symmetrical and a few scattered smaller lesions may also appear on the thighs and extensor aspect of the arms. Occasionally the first lesion is unilateral and forms an extensive plaque of tender erythema which can be mistaken for cellulitis. Rarely lesions of erythema multiforme accompany this eruption.

There are three important causes in Britain, tuberculosis, strepto-coccal infection and sarcoidosis. Their proportions vary according to the age and domicile of the patient.

In Sheffield, 75 per cent of cases in adults are precipitated by a streptococcal sore throat or tonsillitis 10–14 days before the onset of lesions. In children, the number due to primary tuberculous infection is now very small in Britain but is still significant in many other countries. In these cases the lesions appear at or shortly after the time at which sensitivity to tuberculin has been demonstrated to change from negative to positive. In children the majority of cases are caused by streptococcal infection, but it must not be assumed that the history of a preceding sore throat rules out tuberculosis as it is also found in cases of erythema nodosum of definite tuberculous aetiology. In the adult, the number of

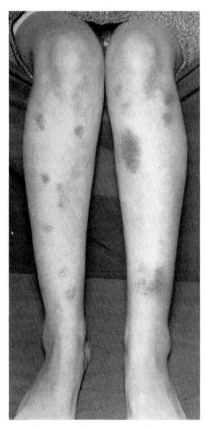

FIG. 59.—Erythema nodosum.

cases of tuberculous aetiology is very small, accounting for less than 10 per cent in a skin clinic, but higher figures may be recorded when there is selection of such cases in a chest clinic.

Sarcoidosis shows such a wide range of incidence in different localities that it can be found to be responsible for one-third of adult cases in Buckinghamshire and for less than 10 per cent in Yorkshire.

Other causes are rare and consist of drug reactions, particularly to sulphathiazole; similar nodules may occur in meningococcal septicaemia though usually smaller; leprosy, especially when under treatment with dapsone, may produce these lesions as a reaction; coccidioidomycosis in areas in South West United States where it is endemic can give rise to similar lesions.

Investigation of the patient reveals a slight rise in the total white cell count with insignificant changes in the differential count. The sedimentation rate is markedly elevated and takes from 2–6 months to return to normal. An X-ray picture should be taken of the chest which may reveal unilateral hilar lymph node enlargement and the primary focus of tuberculosis. In sarcoidosis the chest X-ray can help by showing bilateral hilar node enlargement or there may be miliary, linear or nodular infiltration of the lung fields. The Mantoux test should be performed with 1:10,000 tuberculin as in primary tuberculosis the reaction may be severe; in sarcoidosis lower dilutions provoke no reaction in 50 per cent of patients. The antistreptolysin titre will be raised in cases of streptococcal origin and repeated rising titres provide additional support for the diagnosis. The presence or absence of haemolytic streptococci in throat swabs is not useful evidence, since at the stage of this sensitisation reaction they may have been dispersed by antibiotics and secondly, positive cultures have been obtained from the throats of patients with erythema nodosum who have a definite tuberculous infection. Biopsy of the lesions is of no help in deciding the aetiology and shows a perivasculitis in the upper portion of the subcutaneous tissue with an infiltrate of neutrophils and lymphocytes, these also invade the vessel walls of larger veins and there is marked endothelial proliferation. Older lesions also contain giant cells and foci of epithelioid cells. Sarcoidosis may be also present with additional papular lesions in the skin and biopsy of these is more helpful in showing typical histology of dermal clumps of epithelioid cells.

TREATMENT

The general management of the patient depends on the aetiology which these investigations establish but as far as the skin lesions themselves are concerned, the course of the disease is similar. Individual lesions last less than 2 weeks; the time during which new lesions recur depends on whether the patient is at rest, and if put to bed, new lesions usually cease within 2 weeks. If however the patient has not sought advice and remains ambulant, fresh crops of lesions may appear for a month or more, if lesions recur for more than 6 weeks the diagnosis should be reconsidered. Administration of sulphonamides has been shown to aggravate the lesions and it is our impression that penicillin therapy has the same effect. Sometimes, even when at rest in bed, the temperature is slow to settle to normal; we have observed this in several patients with previous histories of rheumatic fever but in none was there any evidence of reactivation of rheumatism.

Rest in bed with a cradle to take the weight of the bed clothes off the lesions and analgesics if necessary is the treatment of choice. The patient should remain in bed until the lesions have resolved, as too early mobility can provoke another crop. Corticosteroid therapy is, in our opinion, unnecessary and undesirable.

In very mild cases where bed rest is impossible for social reasons, adhesive elastic bandaging may be applied, with the adhesive side outwards, from the toes to the knees then covered with a bandage. This can be left in place for a week at a time and enables the patient to be ambulant without producing oedema of the legs, nevertheless, as much rest as possible should be advised. Recurrences are not uncommon in the streptococcal group if a fresh infection is acquired.

Erythema induratum (Bazin's disease)

This is a rare disease which is important because its most common cause is active tuberculosis and because the lesions resemble severe chilblains.

It occurs on the lower calves in the area of erythrocyanosis; this chilblain-type of circulation seems to be necessary for formation of lesions, possibly because it provides a sufficiently sluggish circulation for the deposition of tubercle bacilli which have frequently been isolated from lesions. Because cold damage of the calves is commoner in young women they are predominantly the sufferers from erythema induratum.

The lesions consist of deeply infiltrated plaques and nodules, cyanotic in colour, cold to touch and symmetrically situated on cold blue areas of the calves. Some of the lesions ulcerate forming deep punched out ulcers about 1–2 cm. in diameter. Chilblains may occur on a similar site but the nodules and plaques which they produce are superficial and do not produce the brawny induration of erythema induratum; if they ulcerate, they do so very shallowly producing little more than a break in the epidermis.

The attack of erythema induratum usually begins in cold weather and lesions fluctuate, often improving and healing with scar formation

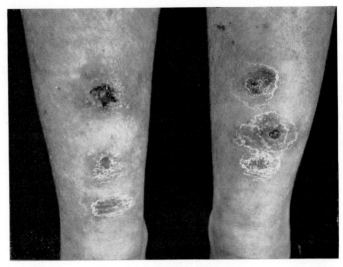

FIG. 60.—Erythema induratum.

in the summer but recurring again with cold weather, making their course even more like chilblains.

In some cases there is a history of tuberculous infection but in others a systematic search may have to be made to trace the site of active disease which may be in the lungs, abdominal lymph nodes, kidneys or bones. Pyrexia, a high sedimentation rate, a strongly positive Mantoux test, and raised gamma globulin are the usual findings in such cases. Chronic streptococcal infection has been incriminated in some cases but so high is the incidence of tuberculosis as the cause of this disease that even if the focus of infection cannot be traced it is advisable to treat the patient with a full antituberculous regime of streptomycin P.A.S. and isoniazid. The skin lesions heal rapidly but until they have healed, reversed elastoplast bandages should be applied to the legs and left in place for a week at a time.

Anaphylactoid purpura

This is an allergic reaction to infection, the most commonly traceable cause being streptococcal. Occasionally drugs such as penicillin may be incriminated but it is difficult to dissociate antibiotic drugs from the infection for which they were prescribed. The protean manifestations of the disease are due to the fact that the basic lesion is a capillaritis which can involve any organ but it is the appearance of skin lesions which establishes the diagnosis.

Anaphylactoid purpura may occur at any age, the classical sequence of streptococcal tonsillitis followed after 10–14 days by the skin lesions and other manifestations is commoner in children. In the adult, the precipitating cause may not be so obvious, nor is the interval between infections and onset so clear cut. In the elderly, chest infection is a common association.

Skin lesions are not necessarily the first manifestation; they consist of urticarial papules 0·5 to 1 cm. in diameter into which is a varying degree of purpura, so that this may appear to be the basic lesion. It is therefore important to notice that these lesions are raised and palpable, unlike thrombocytopenic purpura which produces no alteration in the skin texture. If the degree of purpura is severe enough to produce an ecchymosis the centre of the papule may become necrotic and form a small circinate ulcer with a black slough; gravity increases the purpura and necrotic ulcers are therefore more common on the feet and legs.

The skin lesions may consist of only a few papules on the feet and legs which are of diagnostic help only to the observant, or can be profuse, in which case the thighs, buttocks, arms and extensor aspect of the upper arms are predominantly involved, though scattered lesions may affect the trunk. Hess's test of capillary fragility is negative (except for an increase in purpura in the lesions). The skin lesions tend to recur in crops and in the attack two or three crops during about 6 weeks is the usual course.

Preceding or coinciding with the skin lesions the most common symptom is flitting joint pains sometimes with obvious hydrarthrosis. Any joint may be affected but commonly the wrists, ankles and knees. The patient is usually febrile. Abdominal pain may accompany melaena and in young people appendicitis may be diagnosed if the skin eruption is not noticed. Haematuria and albuminuria denote involvement of the kidneys but it is uncommon for the haematuria to be more than microscopic, despite the fact that kidney biopsy has established that some degree of renal involvement occurs in all cases. The prognosis depends on the degree of kidney involvement, therefore examination for haematuria should be repeated at intervals. Pathological investigation also demonstrates a raised sedimentation rate in most cases and in many a rising antistreptolysin titre suggesting a recent streptococcal infection as the cause.

In acute cases the patient should be kept at rest in bed until the skin lesions cease to appear and until haematuria, if present, has ceased. Systemic corticosteroid therapy should only be used if there is evidence of severe involvement of the kidneys; its effectiveness is doubtful as it has no effect on the skin lesions though it does control the joint symptoms. Continuous oral penicillin is a valuable prophylactic measure in children suffering recurrent attacks associated with tonsillitis.

Rarely the eruption continues in crops for months or years; obviously

bed rest is out of the question in these cases but sometimes cortico-
tropin therapy helps.

Polyarteritis nodosa

This is a further degree of hypersensitivity reaction than those
already described; small arteries and arterioles throughout the body
are involved in localised areas of inflammation, producing nodules.
Circumstantial evidence points to drugs as the most common cause.
In the skin all the eruptions of erythema multiforme, urticaria, purpura
and anaphylactoid-type purpura and erythema nodosum may be
produced, often in a polymorphic eruption. Nodules in the skin formed
by involved arterioles are a useful diagnostic sign and confirmation
can be established by biopsy of such a nodule.

In more chronic cases damage to skin arterioles produces broken
areas of fixed livedo due to capillary stasis.

The acute form of the disease causes a severe febrile illness and
the damage caused by involvement of the arterioles may affect any
system, producing an endless variety of symptoms and signs which
include peripheral neuritis, abdominal pain and melaena, haematuria
and evidence of lung damage. Corticosteroids are the only effective
treatment.

Chronic discoid lupus erythematosus

This is a disease of unknown aetiology which occurs in the third and
fourth decades of life in women more often than men. Usually the
lesions occur on the face in the area of the nose and cheeks, forehead or

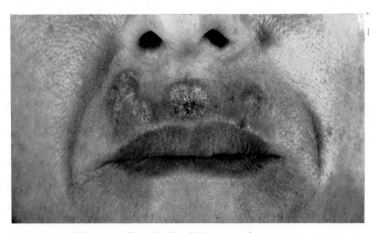

FIG. 61.—Chronic discoid lupus erythematosus.

preauricular area. Symmetry is uncommon and the classical distribution over the "butterfly" area formed by nose and cheeks is rare.

The lesions are sharply demarkated discs of slightly scaly erythema. The degree of thickening and infiltration varies; long standing lesions are scarred in the centre though they may still show active edges. On close examination the follicles are prominent owing to the formation of a keratin plug which is characteristic and can sometimes be demonstrated by peeling off a scale and showing the follicular plugs adhering to its under surface as a brush of spikes. Telangiectases are usual in the lesion and it is important to notice that no translucent nodules are present when the blood is expressed with a glass slide, thus differentiating it from lupus vulgaris. Lesions may occur in the scalp producing loss of hair; when activity ceases a pale scarred area of permanent baldness remains. More widespread discs occur in some cases involving the dorsum or palmar aspect of the fingers. Exposure to sunlight aggravates the patches and can be such an important factor that activity occurs only in the summer months.

Haematological investigation of cases of chronic discoid lupus erythematosus reveals a raised sedimentation rate in about one-third of cases and presence of LE cells in approximately one-fifth; a few cases may show other abnormalities such as leukopenia. However, despite these findings it is extremely rare for typical discoid lupus to progress to subacute or acute systemic lupus erythematosus; the vas majority of patients remain in good health apart from the skin lesions and even these tend to heal over the course of years regardless of treatment.

TREATMENT

There is no specific treatment of chronic discoid erythematosus since the aetiology is unknown. The lesions should be protected from direct sunlight by the wearing of a hat and the application of a light-barrier cream. The application of fluocinolone acetonide or betamethasone valerate ointment to the lesions three times daily is successful in suppressing the majority of lesions; maintenance application is necessary for months once the lesions have healed. If this is unsuccessful, infiltration of the lesion with triamcinolone by injection is successful in those areas where such a measure is not too painful. Chloroquine sulphate 200 mg. three times daily usually heals the lesion if local steroids fail but should be given in courses which are broken in the winter months to avoid toxic effects on the eyes.

Systemic lupus erythematosus is too rare a disease to be described in detail here. Its main presenting features are of an acute or subacute pyrexial illness mainly affecting women in the reproductive period of life. Skin eruptions may be present and the most usual is a blotchy erythema of the face, neck, V area, hands and arms associated with oedema of the face. Toxic alopecia occurs in most cases. Associated with the skin lesion are a variety of systemic signs including polyarthritis, kidney damage, involvement of serous membranes and blood vessels. In addition to the LE cell phenomenon systemic lupus patients produce a number of abnormal serological reactions due to a variety of auto-antibodies which react with different components of body cells and tissues.

Lymphoma and myelosis

Lymphomas are a group of malignant tumours arising usually from multiple foci of the lymphoid reticular system. The lymphomas may be monomorphic and composed of stem cell, reticulum cell or lymphocytic series or they can be polymorphic as in Hodgkin's disease and mycosis fungoides. Leukaemia may be present at some stage in these groups or it may never arise. Myelosis designates tumours of the myeloid system and is nearly always associated with myeloid leukaemia.

Just as the mode of presentation of these diseases varies greatly so do the cutaneous signs, many of which are shared between all groups. Determination of the type of cell involved rests with the pathologist.

Toxic symptoms produce the usual non-specific cutaneous patterns of pruriginous papules, erythema multiforme-like lesions and purpura. Generalised pruritus in the absence of any apparent cutaneous cause may precede signs of Hodgkins disease by months or years and, more rarely, occurs in lymphatic leukaemia. The persistence of such intractable itching in a young adult should be investigated at intervals for the development of lymphoma or hepatic disease.

Rarely Hodgkin's disease gives rise to an acquired form of ichthyosis.

Generalised exfoliative dermatitis may occur in those suffering from widespread chronic eczema and an almost identical clinical picture may be produced by generalised exfoliative psoriasis. In those cases occurring without any history of previous skin disease it is important to exclude the possibility of underlying Hodgkin's disease, lymphatic leukaemia or mycosis fungoides. In this condition the whole of the patient's skin is dusky red, dry and scaling so profusely that a dustpan and brush may be required to sweep up the small pile of scales shed when the patient removes his clothes. The skin over the whole body is oedematous and pits on pressure while the legs are often grossly swollen. Lymph nodes in the axillae and groins are so enlarged that they can be visible. In the elderly, oedema of the face in the inelastic senile skin causes the eyelids to be everted (ectropion) and conjunctivitis results. With the shedding of skin scales there may be severe loss of hair and shedding of nails.

Blood flow to the skin, which as a whole is a very large organ, is so greatly increased that in an elderly patient on the verge of heart failure the strain on the heart may be sufficient to precipitate him into actual failure. The dilated blood vessels in the skin lose their power to contract and thus lose their thermoregulatory function. Heat lost through the skin is so great that the patient can quickly take on the temperature of his surroundings and even in a centrally heated ward can develop a seriously subnormal temperature.

Finally, severe generalised disorder of the skin upsets the function of the gut causing malabsorption of fats, iron and vitamins and

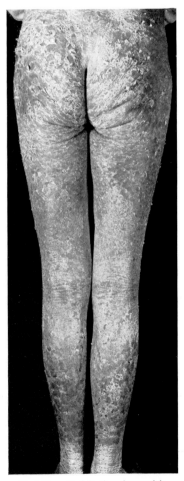

FIG. 62.—Exfoliative dermatitis.

protein loss both from the gut and from the severe scaling of the skin.

Treatment. Large doses of corticosteroids are the only effective treatment of this condition whatever its underlying cause. Before the use of corticosteroids 40 per cent of cases of generalised exfoliative dermatitis died; now the response is rapid and lack of improvement makes the presence of an underlying reticulosis more probable. The temperature of these patients should be taken with a low-reading thermometer so that subnormal temperatures do not pass unnoticed. A side-ward with regulated heating is the most satisfactory way to maintain a normal temperature. A side-ward is also desirable because carriage of pathogenic staphylococci is increased on the damaged skin and it is difficult to prevent particles of scales being carried in the dust through an open ward, carrying with them bacteria and the risks of infection to other patients.

Because of protein loss diet should be high in protein content and supplemented with protein feeds such as "Complan" and with vitamins. If ectropion occurs liquid paraffin drops should be instilled into the eyes to lubricate them several times daily.

Interference with blood cell formation and resistance to infection produces another motley collection of signs. Purpura may be associated with thrombocytopenia, in which case Hess's test will be positive. Furunculosis can be a presenting symptom especially in myeloid leukaemia, boils failing to heal because of infiltration with leukaemia cells so that painful ulcerated nodules are formed. Herpes zoster is a relatively frequent occurrence in the lymphomas, especially in Hodgkin's disease and lymphatic leukaemia. In such cases a generalised chicken-pox like eruption accompanies the localised zoster and this development should be an indication for investigation for underlying disease.

Infiltrations of the skin occur in all groups and consist of nodules and plaques; the nature of the infiltrate can only be determined by biopsy. Infiltration of the skin is rare in Hodgkins disease and usually breaks down to produce painful intractable ulceration. Large nodules in elderly people are often due to reticulum cell lymphomata. Reddish brown profuse translucent nodules in those over 45 years of age may be due to lymphatic leukaemia, but in the same age group an identical appearance can be produced by carcinomatosis.

Mycosis fungoides is a cutaneous syndrome produced by a pleomorphic infiltrate similar to Hodgkin's disease. Infiltration of the skin and tumour formation are the final stages of this lymphoma and are preceded by a variety of non-specific eczematous or psoriasiform eruptions whose severe itching and lack of response to treatment suggest the ultimate development of mycosis though this may not become apparent for years.

One pattern of eruption which is easier to identify as a possible precursor of mycosis fungoides is known as parapsoriasis en plaques. This presents in the adult as slightly scaly brownish red macules which may be isolated, or coalesce into figurate patterns. Once formed they

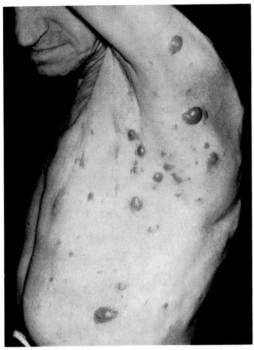

FIG. 63.—Reticulum cell lymphoma.

remain completely resistant to treatment and development into mycosis fungoides can take place after many years. The final pattern produced is a mixture of lesions of parapsoriasis, areas of infiltration of the skin and ulcerated exuding nodules 2–4 cm. in diameter.

Malignant disease

The commonest cutaneous lesions produced by internal carcinomata are nodules in the skin due to secondary deposits. Their nature may be guessed from the age and symptoms of the patient and determination of their source can usually be established by examination of biopsy material.

Rare toxic eruptions occur in association with carcinomata and can resemble pemphigoid in producing bullae, can mimic the fixed lesions of lupus erythematosus or produce a gyrate erythema on the trunk, therefore the possibility of underlying malignant disease should be considered in any unusual eruption in patients over 45 years of age. Dermatomyositis is also precipitated by malignant disease in about 20 per cent of cases above middle age, though it occurs without this association in younger age groups. The condition presents with muscle weakness and wasting caused by inflammatory changes in the muscles. Associated with this is an acute erythema of the light exposed areas of the face and arms, oedema of the face and especially of the eyelids which assume a characteristic violet colour, a streaky erythema over the tendons on the dorsum of the hands and telangiectasia of the nail beds.

CHAPTER 13

PRURITUS

THE sensation of itching is conveyed from the sub-epidermal plexus
of nerves via the pain paths in the antero-lateral tracts of the cord. The
manner in which the nervous system distinguishes between pain or
itching travelling in the same pathway is not fully understood, but is
probably dependent on the periodicity of the impulses. Recent experimental work has shown that proteolytic enzymes can initiate itching
and it is probable that proteases released in small amounts by damage
to epidermal cells accounts for itching in the absence of visible lesions.

A distinction has been made between spontaneous itching which
arises when a new lesion such as an eczema vesicle is formed and the
state of itchiness which is present in many areas of skin inflammation.
In the latter condition, any trivial stimulus such as a light touch can
initiate a paroxysm of itching.

There is great variation in individual capacity to feel itching, some
patients hardly noticing an extensive dermatitis, whilst others suffer
greatly from an eruption which is usually non-pruritic, and even in one
patient, the threshold of itching varies with his state of concentration,
tiredness or boredom. There are also differences in the methods of
scratching for the relief of itching. In atopic eczema and papular
urticaria, scratching with the finger nails until blood is drawn is the
usual method of obtaining relief, whereas in urticaria rubbing with the
finger pads relieves the itching and if excoriations are present this makes
the diagnosis of urticaria less likely.

Generalised itching

Generalised itching, which is more marked in the evenings and in
bed, is a common complaint. Having excluded parasitic diseases such
as scabies and infestation with body lice, there remain a number of
patients in whom no skin abnormality other than excoriations can be
found. Though psychogenic irritation does occur, it is a dangerous
diagnosis to make until the organic disorders, which present with
itching, have been excluded by careful examination and, if necessary,
laboratory investigations. Causes which should be sought are anaemia,
uraemia, liver disease and systemic neoplasms and reticuloses. Normal
urine, blood sugar and blood urea will exclude diabetes and uraemia.
A complete blood count will be needed to eliminate leukaemia and
severe anaemia. Serum iron estimation is of value as pruritis may be
caused when this is low.

More difficult to diagnose is itching due to hepatitis, which may not be accompanied by jaundice. Liver function tests and liver biopsy may be necessary to establish the cause.

Generalised itching may also precede overt evidence of Hodgkin's disease by several years. This possibility must always be kept in mind in the young adult with intractable pruritus and a watch should be kept for superficial lymph gland enlargement and hilar lymph nodes. It may be possible to demonstrate abdominal glands by lymphangiography.

Senile pruritis

This is the most frequent cause of generalised itching in the elderly who often complain of intense itching, particularly on the back between the scapulae, yet on examination no abnormality, not even excoriations, can be found. It is probable that the heightened sensation of itchiness is a result of vascular changes in the cutaneous nerves as it is often associated with generalised arteriosclerosis, but the exact cause is unknown. The elderly also suffer from dryness and scaling of the skin, which can give rise to irritation. This dryness is accentuated by the degreasing effect of soap, if the habit of daily bathing is continued into old age. A similar condition occurring particularly in cold weather in younger age groups is termed winter itch. Senile pruritis may be complicated by dermatitis from self treatment and occasionally the symptoms are ascribed by the patient to parasitic infestation.

Treatment. The natural grease of the skin should be conserved by the restriction of bathing and the addition of emulsifying ointment or Oilatum Emollient to the bath water.

1% Phenol in emulsifying ointment or 3% liquor picis carbonis in aqueous ointment or Boots E. 45 cream are clean and effective anti-pruritic and emollient applications. Lotions should be avoided, since they dry the skin and aggravate the symptoms. Explanations and re-assurance plays a significant part in the relief of irritation, which may be helped by Tab. chlorpromazine hydrochloride, (Largactil) 25 mg. 3 times a day. Androgenic hormones have been advocated but we have seen little benefit from their use.

Pruritus of pregnancy

A number of so called "toxic" eruptions develop in the last three months of pregnancy. Usually itching is accompanied by an urticarial or an erythema multiforme—like rash, but both generalised and localised pruritus can occur without a visible skin change. Anxiety about the significance of the rash and loss of sleep produce considerable mental tension which increases the symptoms.

Reassurance that the eruption does not indicate any harm to the child and that the symptoms will clear after parturition, is of more benefit than local application, but calamine lotion with 1% phenol gives temporary symptomatic relief. Oral progesterone in the form of norethisterone 10 mg. twice daily relieved itching and rash in 80 per cent of cases in a recent report. Once in 4,500 pregnancies, herpes gestationis, a bullous irritable eruption, occurs and this can be controlled only by corticosteroids.

Prurigo

This is a descriptive term for the changes in the skin which are a result of scratching and excoriation. Small, firm papules, crusts and pitted scars occur in papular urticaria, neurotic excoriations, atopic eczema, sunlight eruptions, pregnancy, old age and generalised pruritus of systemic origin. It is not a disease entity.

Localised pruritus

The commonest site for intractable localised itching is the anogenital region. Other sites have been mentioned under lichen simplex (page 39). To a great extent, the state of itchiness is due to a heightened awareness of sensation with the result that any slight stimulus is sufficient to initiate a paroxysm of itching and scratching. This damages the skin further and strengthens the conditioned reflex. Sufferers from localised pruritus are tense, excitable people but it should be remembered that intense and chronic itching may alter the mental state of an individual. Thus itching of organic origin may transform the placid, equable tempered into aggressive, complaining individuals in a remarkably short time.

Pruritus of the anogenital region has, in addition, a sexual connotation, some deriving pleasure from stimuli in this way and others using the disorder as an excuse for the refusal of sexual intercourse. Another factor is cancerphobia and, unless directly questioned, many patients will not voice their fears. There are therefore in every case both organic and psychogenic components which must be elicited by an adequate history and examination.

Pruritus ani

As has been mentioned previously, a heightened awareness of sensations is necessary for them to reach the conscious level and pruritus ani is often started by some organic lesion such as a tear in the mucosa, a fissure in ano or often an operation for haemorrhoids. Discharge from the rectum, either because of piles, proctitis or a leaking sphincter or diarrhoea may initiate itching by the production of maceration of the perianal skin. Contact dermatitis due to medicaments, particularly local anaesthetic ointments, is a common cause which may mask any underlying factor. Contact dermatitis due to toilet paper or clothing is a possibility but not a frequent offender. Local skin lesions of psoriasis, seborrhoeic intertrigo, lichen planus and ringworm may be found. Ringworm should be suspected if there are active lesions between the toes, which should always be examined. A common cause is recent treatment with broad spectrum antibiotics which allow *Candida* to increase in the intestine and spread to the perianal skin. The infestation with threadworms is often responsible for pruritus ani in children but rarely in adults. The diagnosis can be confirmed by detection of the ova on the skin around the anus. When all these causes have been excluded, a considerable number of patients will remain in whom either no abnormality can be found or, at most, slight excoriations of the perianal skin. In some, the irritation may be associated with sweating, but in many no organic explanation can be found. It is this group which deserve investigation of psychogenic factors, though symptomatic relief can be obtained by local treatment.

Treatment. The patient should be exhorted to resist the temptation to scratch, and stimuli to the perianal region should be reduced as much as possible. Cotton wool or soft paper tissue must be substituted for toilet paper. Many patients are obsessional about cleanliness and over-use of soap and particularly antiseptics must be avoided. A topical steroid ointment applied 3 times daily will produce relief in a high proportion of patients but atrophy follows prolonged use of penetrating steroids and they should be reserved for the treatment of psoriasis and seborrhoeic intertrigo. If *Candida* is suspected, an ointment which also contains an antiseptic such as iodochlorhydroxyquinoline (Vioform) and nystatin is to be preferred. Any surgical abnormality should be corrected but not until local irritation has been controlled. Ringworm infection responds well to Castellani's paint but griseofulvin may be needed in resistant cases. Once the pruritus is under control, applications of steroid ointment should be reduced slowly, but treatment may need to be prolonged for many months to prevent recurrence.

Pruritus vulvae

As with anal irritation, the itching may be caused by maceration of the skin from discharge which can be due to *Candida* or trichomonal infection of the vagina. Pregnancy and diabetes and the use of broad spectrum antibiotics all precipitate an acute candidiasis. The vivid red intertrigo of the vulva and groins with outlying vesico-pustules is a clinical picture which should indicate immediately a test for glycosuria. Contact dermatitis caused by medicaments is always common and the possibility of sensitivity to rubber and chemical contraceptives should not be forgotten. As in the natal cleft, so the groins and vulva may be affected by psoriasis, seborrhoea and lichen planus, but ringworm is a rarity in women.

Pediculosis pubis should be considered and excluded. The presence of the lice and ova on the hairs can be easily overlooked unless a conscious effort to search for them is made. Itching associated with a white thickening of the vulval mucosa and skin is a common problem and a similar clinical picture is produced by three different conditions which has led to much confusion and dissention between dermatologists and gynaecologists:

(i) *Lichen simplex of the vulva.* This is a result of prolonged scratching due probably to a psychogenic cause. Lichenification usually involves the labia majora as well as the labia minora but sodden white keratinisation of the mucosa can resemble leucoplakia and may only be distinguishable by biopsy. If irritation can be controlled by topical steroid ointment, the white thickened areas of lichenification disappear, whereas leucoplakia remains unchanged.

(ii) *Lichen sclerosus.* This condition is a disorder of collagen allied to scleroderma. There is a well defined, shiny, atrophic change in the skin over the clitoris and labia minora and lesions often extend backwards to the perianal region. Plaques of lichen sclerosus may also be found on the thighs and other parts of the body. The line of demarcation between diseased skin and the normal is very clear. The surface of the affected skin is rough and shows horny plugs and telangiectases. Itching commonly arises from infection and fissuring of the inelastic surface. Lichen sclerosus may be complicated by leucoplakia.

(iii) *Leucoplakia.* This is a premalignant change which may arise on the vulval mucosa which otherwise shows no atrophy or inflammation or it may be superimposed on a pre-existing disorder. Diagnosis in the latter is impossible without continued observation and biopsy. The irregular, hard, thickened plaques of leucoplakia are intensely irritable.

Treatment. The general approach to treatment should be similar to that for anal pruritus and any sort of vaginal discharge given the requisite treatment. Obviously, if diabetes is present, it must be controlled. Creams active against *Candida* such as nystatin are indicated if candidiasis is present. Any underlying cause of emotional tension should be discussed and anxiety and sleeplessness controlled by sedation. The changes of lichen sclerosus may persist for many years but some cases recover completely. Symptoms may be alleviated by topical steroids. Patients with lichen sclerosus must be kept under observation every 2 to 3 months since leucoplakia and malignant change may complicate the condition. Most authorities do not consider the risk is so great initially that vulvectomy is indicated but inability to relieve itching suggests that leucoplakia is more likely to occur ultimately. Once the diagnosis of true leucoplakia is established vulvectomy is indicated since carcinoma follows in 50 per cent of cases.

CHAPTER 14

PSORIASIS

PSORIASIS and its treatment form a major problem in dermatology. The incidence of the disorder in the general population is calculated to be about 1 to 2 per cent, it appears for the first time between the ages of 5 and 25 years in the majority of patients. Once established remissions are uncommon and brief—only about 10 per cent of sufferers being free from all traces of psoriasis for more than 5 years at a time. Girls suffering from psoriasis outnumber boys by 2 to 1 but by the time adult life is reached about 40 per cent of cases are male and there is no difference in the severity of the disease in either sex.

Aetiology. Although the cause is unknown there are several factors which influence its onset, the most important of which is heredity. The incidence of a family history of the disease may vary in different regions depending probably on variations in stability of the population and the resultant differences in inbreeding. In Yorkshire about 33 per cent of psoriatics can trace another similarly affected member of the family. In areas of static population and inbreeding psoriasis may appear in many generations affecting several siblings and in such families the condition tends to be severe and persistent. In a disease which may appear at any age and whose stigmata may be so slight as to pass unnoticed, it is difficult to work out the mode of inheritance, but it appears to be one of irregular dominance in most cases, though sometimes recessive. The risk of psoriasis for children of one affected parent is 25 per cent; for siblings of an affected child with normal parents 17 per cent; for siblings of an affected child with one affected parent 30 per cent.

Another factor which may influence the onset of psoriasis is infection, streptococcal tonsillitis in childhood being the precipitating cause of 50 per cent of acute cases of psoriasis of the widespread guttate pattern in childhood. In patients with the chronic pattern of psoriasis a streptococcal upper respiratory infection may precipitate an exacerbation of the disease. Such an infection is followed by an interval of 10 to 14 days before the onset or flare of the psoriasis suggesting an allergic response to infection as the trigger factor and very rarely one may see another allergic response such as acute nephritis appearing at the same time. Deprivation of sunlight must also play some part in influencing the disease. In sunny climates it is not common in white races and the low incidence in dark skinned races may be partly geographic rather than due to racial differences in incidence. There is however a higher incidence among the races of Northern Europe and a noticeable fluctuation in the disease with the seasons, most psoriatics improving in the summer months. The response of the disease to tropical and subtropic climates depends on its severity. Those with very extensive psoriasis are likely to become worse as the result of sweating and maceration of the skin if exposed to extreme heat and

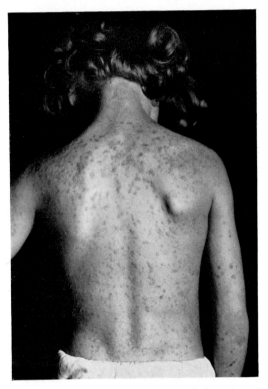

Fig. 64.—Acute guttate psoriasis.

humidity. Those with mild lesions often clear completely in subtropical or tropical countries and remain clear until they return to their native lack of sunshine.

Mental stress is not a common factor in precipitating the first attack of psoriasis, though occasional patients give such a convincingly close history of stress and onset of the disease that it cannot be discounted. It is also supported by the undoubted influence which stress has over the course of established psoriasis, as relapses in extent of the lesions are not uncommon as the result of worry or shock.

The course is also influenced by hormonal factors, commencing or
becoming worse with puberty or at the menopause and often improving
during pregnancy. Whether the condition has altered during pregnancy or not it usually relapses after childbirth. Despite these

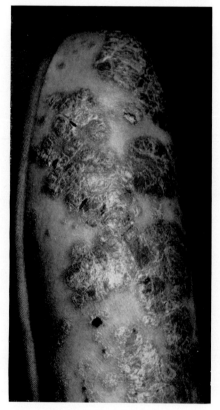

Fig. 65.—Chronic psoriasis.

influences there is no evidence that psoriasis is caused by hormonal
factors.

Clinical features. The lesions of psoriasis consist of sharply
demarcated red or pink areas of skin with silvery scaling which may
become heaped up on the affected areas. If scaling is not obvious the
characteristic silvery colour of the scales appears when the lesion is
scratched, scratching causing separation of surface scales and allowing
air between them to reflect back the light. Further scratching separates
the scaly layer from a velvety red epidermis in which bleeding points

appear where the tips of the papillae and the capillaries have been damaged.

The pattern, distribution and extent of these lesions varies greatly. In an acute attack of psoriasis, which is commoner in childhood and often precipitated by infection, the lesions are tiny discs, described as guttate, scattered evenly over the body and limbs, usually also in the

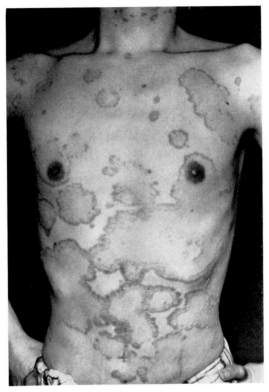

FIG. 66.—Psoriasis.

scalp and sometimes on the face. Unlike pityriasis rosea, the lesions are round rather than oval and do not show the patterning of the lines of cleavage of the skin. When it appears in childhood this acute attack usually clears spontaneously in 2 or 3 months but most of these children will later develop a chronic pattern of psoriasis and in half of them this will appear within 5 years. Infection may similarly produce a guttate attack of lesions in adults who have established chronic psoriasis.

Chronic lesions classically appear as plaques on the knees and elbows, a solitary lesion of this type may pass unrecognised or even unnoticed for years. Other characteristic areas are over the sacrum and in the scalp. The scalp lesions remain as sharply demarcated as those on the rest of the skin and as the scales tend to be anchored by hair they may accumulate considerably so that the lesions can be located by touch. They differ from seborrhoeic dermatitis in that this produces a diffuse scaly erythema extending to the hair margin without much heaping of scales. Fortunately, hair loss does not occur in the affected areas of the scalp unless the lesions are itchy and hair is rubbed off when scratching.

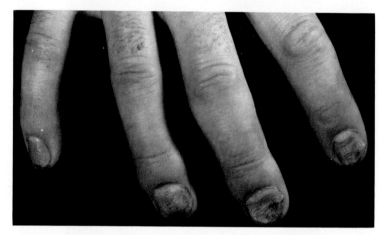

Fig. 67.—Psoriasis of the nails.

Other plaques of varying size and pattern may appear anywhere on the trunk and limbs, often producing remarkably symmetrical lesions in a mirror image pattern; sometimes large sheets, sometimes discs or annular lesions which revert to normal skin in the centres.

In some cases these sheets may spread rapidly, often as the result of maltreatment, until they coalesce to cover every inch of the body producing a picture indistinguishable from exfoliative dermatitis. The history of the state of the skin before generalisation of the eruption differentiates the conditions; clinically there is less oedema of the skin in exfoliative psoriasis and reactive lymph node enlargement is not a feature.

Involvement of the finger nails occurs in about a quarter of all cases and is sometimes seen as the only manifestation of psoriasis. Pitting resembling that on a thimble is the commonest change, but either in association with this or alone, the nails may be ridged transversely and scales heap up under the ends of the nails, producing thickened opaque

and discoloured nails which, with severe involvement, become broken
or loose and severely malformed.

Lesions may appear in the axillae, groins and umbilicus which,
because of the moist situation, do not become scaly and may even
exude serum. In these areas psoriasis maintains its sharply demarcated
edge which differentiates it from seborrhoeic dermatitis or moniliasis.

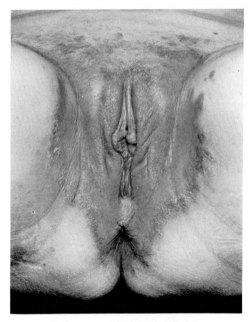

FIG. 68.—Flexural psoriasis.

Flexural lesions can occur at any age but are a special feature of psoriasis
in middle aged women at or beyond the menopause; a careful search
for other manifestations of psoriasis usually reveals the true nature of
the lesion.

Alteration of the usual appearances of the lesions on the palms and
soles can lead to difficulties in diagnosis. Small scaly discs may be
scattered over the palms, these usually also affect the knuckles and give
rise to much discomfort by their tendency to fissure. Sometimes these
hyperkeratotic discs may coalesce to form one large hyperkeratotic
area over the palms or soles which is usually itchy. In addition to
redness and scaling, pustules may appear on palms and soles situated
deep in the epidermis; because of the toughness of the horny layer
these do not rupture, but resolve leaving yellow thickenings of the

epidermis which eventually are desquamated. In the absence of other lesions of psoriasis, pustular lesions are difficult to differentiate from the pustular lesions found in recurrent pomphloyx of the palms and soles or some cases of eczema of palms and soles, chronicity and resistance to treatment being more of a feature in pustular psoriasis.

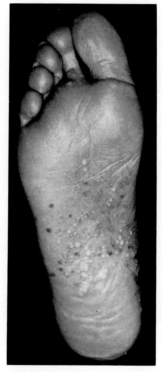

FIG. 69.—Pustular psoriasis.

Arthropathy. Psoriasis is sufficiently common for it to appear in conjunction with rheumatoid arthritis and osteoarthritis in many cases. There is however a type of psoriatic arthropathy which seems to be a separate entity.

The incidence in sufferers from psoriasis is low and although about 7 per cent occur amongst hospital patients the onset of arthritis makes hospital attendance more likely. Any joints may be affected but the most typical are the interphalangeal joints and the lumbar spine. The terminal interphalangeal joints are usually involved as opposed to the proximal interphalangeal joints in rheumatoid arthritis and almost invariably the affected fingers show nail changes. X-rays show erosive changes in the affected areas and the Rose Waaler test, which is positive in 80 per cent of cases of rheumatoid arthritis, is negative in psoriatic arthropathy. It is not common for this type of arthritis to progress to severe deformity, though very rarely absorbtion of the phalanges may produce "concertina-like" changes in the fingers.

The course of psoriasis is so variable, the disfigurement it produces so distressing and its response to psychogenic factors so marked that it lends itself to quack therapies whose worth is disproportionate to their expense. For this reason medical practitioners should maintain an optimistic approach to treatment as although permanent cure is not possible, very much can be done to ameliorate the condition.

Patients looking back on a lifetime of psoriasis can often recall periods of months or years when the disease was extensive and distressing. Puberty, the late teens and early twenties and the menopause are the ages of stress when psoriasis, in common with many other skin complaints, may flare up, but often there are long intervals between when a few patches on knees and elbows are the only trace.

Pathogenesis. The histological changes are those which one would expect in a lesion which daily produces quantities of scale; the horny layer is increased and the cells retain degenerate nuclei instead of forming amorphous keratin. The whole epidermis is thickened in the lesions and there is increased mitotic activity. In radioisotope studies it has been shown that the time for epidermal replacement in the plaque is 3 or 4 days as compared with about 28 days for normal skin. In the dermis there is a cellular infiltrate and a characteristic feature is the dilatation of capillaries high in the dermis which on capillary microscopy have a tortuosity which has been likened to glomeruli.

Associated with the increased cellular activity in the plaques there are metabolic and enzymic changes, but these can also be demonstrated to a lesser degree in the normal skin of the psoriatic subject and the capillary changes can also be observed in the psoriatic's clinically unaffected skin.

TREATMENT

Acute guttate psoriasis subsides spontaneously and sometimes completely in 2 to 3 months. At the stage of eruption it is easily irritated by local applications or ultraviolet light and treatment should be confined to a simple bland application such as 4% liquor picis carb. in aqueous ointment B.P. for a few weeks until the lesions become static, after which it can be treated in the same way as chronic psoriasis.

Many patients with chronic psoriasis respond quite dramatically to local applications only. They should be instructed to soak at night in a warm bath and scrub the scales off the lesions with a soft nail brush.

After drying the skin coal tar and salicylic acid ointment B.P.C. is rubbed into the lesions and they are then covered with stockinette or "Tubegauze" to keep the ointment off the clothes. If tar applications do not help, dithranol may be applied in a base of zinc paste as this prevents the medicament running onto normal skin. A start should be made with $\frac{1}{4}\%$ dithranol but if the surrounding skin is not irritated the concentration can be increased gradually to 5% if necessary. In very thick, scaly, plaques which tend to crack dithranol is better tolerated in a base of yellow soft paraffin in higher concentrations than in a paste. Dithranol stains the skin round the lesions black; as desquamation in the lesion ceases this too takes up the stain as an indication that resolution has occurred. Dithranol should not be used in the flexures as there is a risk of folliculitis, or on the face where the more sensitive skin is easily irritated, in these areas triamcinolone or fluocetonide ointments penetrate the skin sufficiently well to control most cases.

If the lesions are scanty and the patient objects to the greasiness of ointments, pigmentum picis carb. B.P. is useful and if allowed to dry before dressing does not soil the clothes.

Psoriasis of the scalp is more difficult to control and requires conscientious application. The scalp should be washed in 1–2% Cetrimide (Cetavlon) nightly or as often as possible, after which in mild cases a lotion of liquor picis carb., spirit and water in equal parts or 2–4% liquor picis carb. in aqueous ointment B.P. applied to the scalp. In cases where scaling is more severe the messy application of Ung. pyrogallol co. after washing is the only really effective treatment. The hair should be parted in turn from one side of the scalp to the other and the ointment applied to the scalp so that the hair is not matted down.

If local applications do not help the most useful adjunct is ultraviolet light therapy. Suberythema doses 3 times weekly are of considerable value and local treatment with ointment is continued while this is given. The skin pigments in about 6 weeks and after this there is little further improvement. A modification of the Goeckerman regime using the light sensitising effect of tar gives very much better results: the patient soaks for 10 minutes in a warm bath to which liquor picis carbonis has been added (120 ml. in 90 litres of water). Scaly lesions are scrubbed with a soft nail brush. After drying the patient is exposed to ultraviolet light for a suberythema dose, the time of exposure being increased by 30 seconds each day. The lesions are then anointed with coal tar and salicylic acid ointment and the limbs and trunk covered with stockinette. This process takes half-an-hour each day and the patient can then return to work. Mild cases may clear after 3 weeks of this treatment but severe cases require up to 6 weeks. About a third of patients clear completely and all except about 10 per cent derive great benefit, lesions remaining being minimal. In

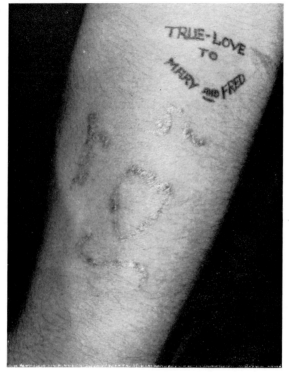

FIG. 70.—Koebner phenomenon in psoriasis.

patients with very extensive psoriasis treatment by the same method in hospital may be preferable and then it is rare for it not to clear completely, sometimes in two to three weeks.

Systemic therapies which are known to affect the eruption all have the disadvantage of toxicity. The only corticosteroid which has any definite effect on psoriasis when given by mouth is triamcinolone but any suppressive effect it may have soon diminishes and psoriasis reappears if the drug is continued or relapses with redoubled spread if the drug is stopped. Systemic corticosteroids should not be used in the treatment of uncomplicated psoriasis. Because of the increased mitotic activity in the lesions antimitotic drugs have been used in treatment for 20 years and the drug commonly prescribed is the folic acid antagonist methotrexate. This is usually given orally and there are advocates of various regimes, one routine being 2.5 mg. daily for 4 to 5 days followed by 3 to 4 days rest. Methotrexate is undoubtedly effective but its toxic effects severely limit its use. It should not be given in the reproductive period of life for fear of teratogenic effects. It may depress bone marrow activity to a dangerous degree and thus frequent routine blood counts are necessary. In a few patients even a small dose can suppress activity in the lesions to such an extent that they necrose and leave large raw areas. Finally, a number of patients have developed cirrhosis of the liver after prolonged treatment with this drug and, as it has been shown to concentrate in the liver, it is unlikely that varied schedules or dosage would prevent this. It is therefore a drug to be used only for incapacitating psoriasis and under close hospital supervision.

Hydrocortisone applied to the skin has no effect on psoriasis but the more powerful fluocinolone acetonide or betamethasone valerate ointments suppress psoriasis of the flexures and face. Applied at night under a sheet of polythene to make the psoriatic area airtight, chronic lesions on limbs and trunk resolve in about a week. This treatment has no effect on psoriasis in the acute or eruptive stage, and when application stops the lesions often recur within a week or two, maintenance therapy without occlusion usually being necessary. Folliculitis under the polythene is a complicating side effect but is less common if the lesions are occluded only at night rather than for longer periods. Expense and rapidity of relapse, sometimes with rebound spread of lesions make the treatment of doubtful value in extensive psoriasis but it is useful for chronic localised lesions and in pustular psoriasis of the palms and soles which usually resist other treatments.

X-ray therapy has no place in the management of ordinary psoriasis but is occasionally useful in flexural psoriasis in post-menopausal women.

Once psoriasis is clear the question of preventing recurrence arises. In acute psoriasis following tonsillitis, especially if this has recurred more than once, tonsillectomy may be considered, but the tonsils should only be removed on their own merit, as the influence on the future course of psoriasis is doubtful.

After ultraviolet light therapy the period of freedom from lesions varies from a few weeks to years, but in most patients fresh lesions appear in an average of 6 months. The use of an ultraviolet lamp at home as a prophylactic measure may lengthen the remission but will do little to influence the relapse when it does occur.

CHAPTER 15

PITYRIASIS ROSEA AND LICHEN PLANUS

Pityriasis rosea

The commonest cause of a slightly itchy eruption of acute onset in a young person which lasts over a week is pityriasis rosea. In many cases the history alone suggests the diagnosis as the condition starts with a solitary lesion commonly found in the scapular area or lower abdomen, oval in shape, slightly scaly and red. Three or four days later an eruption appears which, within a few days, involves most of the trunk. This should be viewed from a distance, preferably by daylight and it will be seen to form a pattern on the trunk in that the macules, which are one of its components, are arranged with their long axis in the lines of cleavage of the skin which correspond roughly to the lines of the ribs in the thorax and transverse lines in the abdominal and lumbar areas. Involving the trunk mainly, it usually ceases on the upper thighs and upper arms and is thus described as confined to the vest and pants area.

Closer inspection reveals that there are two components, pink papules and oval macules, the proportion of which varies; when papules predominate the diagnosis may be more difficult. The configuration of the macules is often best preserved on the flanks where rubbing and scratching is less. Usually 2 to 3 cm. in their long axis they have a pink areola and a fawn coloured centre. At the margin of the fawn area there is scaling which is characteristically centripetal. There is no systemic disturbance apart from itching which varies from slight to severe in different patients and there are no other physical signs.

This is the classical picture of pityriasis rosea which is easy to diagnose, but there are variations on this theme. In the first place the herald patch may remain the only sign for anything up to four weeks before the generalised rash appears. Usually the face and neck are spared but when the neck is involved the macules coalesce to form a reticular scaly eruption which, if it extends to the face, becomes a confluent scaly erythema. In the later stages of the eruption it commonly extends down the arms and legs as it fades on the trunk but, occasionally, the arms and legs are predominantly involved from the onset and sometimes macules may also appear on the palms. Rarely the macules are so large that they are mistaken for ringworm.

The differential diagnosis is important as it is such a common problem. Tinea pedis may produce a sensitisation eruption consisting of macules very like pityriasis rosea but usually more pronounced on the

limbs. In such cases the tinea will be sufficiently active to be obvious
if looked for.

Seborrhoeic dermatitis may give rise to a macular eruption on the
trunk but this is usually scattered at random, without the patterning
of pityriasis rosea; other stigmata of the seborrhoeic state accompany it,
such as scurfy scalp, otitis externa, blepharitis and flexural intertrigo.

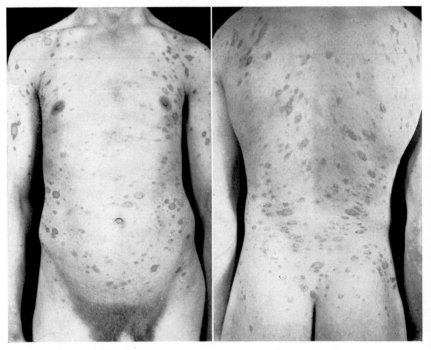

FIG. 71 (a).—Pityriasis rosea.   FIG. 71 (b).—Pityriasis rosea.

In the end persistence for longer than is usual with pityriasis rosea may
be the main clue.

Guttate psoriasis often starts after a sore throat and the lesions are
dotted at random over limbs and trunk. They are uniformly scaly and
round rather than oval; the scalp is frequently involved and here
palpable scaly discs are produced.

Secondary syphilis should always be in one's mind in such a differential diagnosis, even though it is now rare. The usual macular eruption is best seen in daylight and does not have the pattern of the
macule of pityriasis rosea even though it may have a similar colour. Its
ridistbution is universal and more marked scaly lesions occur on palms

and soles. Concomitant signs such as snail track ulcers of the buccal mucosa, generalised lymphadenopathy, condyloma lata of the genitalia, perianal area and other flexures and sometimes the scar of the primary sore reveal the diagnosis, but the Wassermann and Kahn reactions should be performed in any case where this diagnosis is even faintly possible.

The cause of pityriasis rosea is unknown; the herald patch followed by a generalised rash which attacks the young and does not usually recur suggests an infection such as a virus, but so far there is no confirmation.

The eruption lasts about 6 weeks from the time of generalisation; in some it may disappear more quickly, in others it may spread down the arms and legs as it clears on the trunk and take anything up to 12 weeks before it has completely resolved.

Treatment. Many patients suffer so little discomfort that no treatment need be given other than advice to avoid too hot baths, which cause itching. Others itch violently and can be relieved by application of calamine lotion with 1% phenol and an antipruritic drug such as promethazine (Phenergan) mgms. 50 at night. If there is any special urgency for the eruption to be cleared, ultraviolet light therapy in suberythema doses three times weekly is worth trying though not always effective.

Lichen planus

The sufferer from lichen planus usually complains of an itching eruption of sudden onset, starting on the wrists and spreading to trunk and legs. Once established its course is prolonged and by the time advice is sought the rash may have been present for weeks or months.

The skin should be examined by daylight if possible and it will be found that the papular eruption tends to involve the flexural aspect of

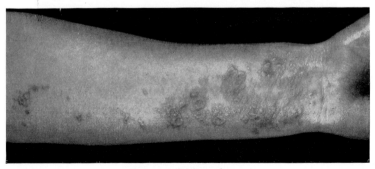

Fig. 72.—Lichen planus.

the wrists and forearms, the trunk and the shins. In a severe attack it may spread beyond these areas or in a mild attack may only present a few lesions on wrists or shins.

The individual lesions are highly characteristic, consisting of purplish, flat topped, shiny papules, polygonal in outline and often umbilicated.

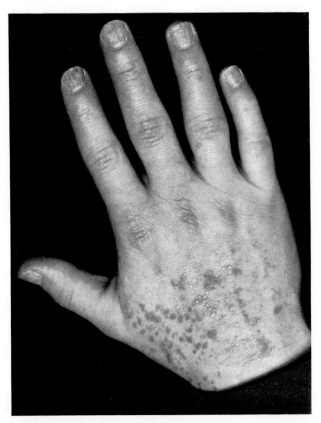

FIG. 73.—Lichen planus showing papules and nail involvement.

Papules frequently occur in scratch marks (Koebner's phenomenon). A magnified lesion can be seen to have the purplish colour broken by a network of Wickham's striae which are delicate white lines. The histological changes of lichen planus are hyperkeratosis and a patchy increase in thickness of the stratum granulosum, a band like infiltrate of mainly lymphocytes hugging the epidermis and irregular acanthosis giving rise to a saw-tooth appearance of the papillae. On the shins the lesions become warty, larger and form plaques which still retain the characteristic colour.

In very severe cases the papules are so numerous that they coalesce, giving the affected areas a solidly purplish colour and, very rarely, small tense vesicles may appear. On palms and soles the colour change is less evident and the papules appear as rather translucent lesions resembling vesicles but hard and hyperkeratotic. In more chronic cases the lesions on the trunk assume an annular pattern.

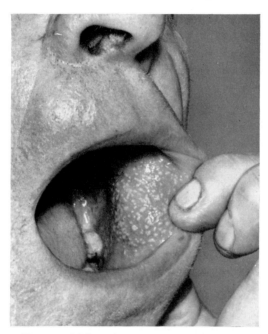

FIG. 74.—Lichen planus of the buccal mucosa.

Mouth lesions are an important aid to diagnosis and may occur in the absence of any skin lesions. They can be present at the onset of the eruption, arise during its course or never appear at all. Delicate white striae on the buccal mucosa opposite the premolar teeth are commonest, but they can be annular lesions or profuse white dots, resembling moniliasis but immovable. Similar lesions may appear on the tongue and white striae appear on the red margin of the lip. Indolent ulcers occur in a few cases, which tend to protrude a plateau of granulation tissue flecked with yellow exudate; the edges of the ulcer, still showing white striae, may also be scarred. Such ulceration occurs at the sides of the tongue and on the buccal mucosa, it is uncomfortable and tender but not acutely painful like aphthous ulcers. Like all chronic inflammatory lesions of mucocutaneous junctions these ulcers are potentially malignant and the incidence of epitheliomata has been put as high as 20 per cent. In such a site epitheliomata grow rapidly and mouth ulceration should be reviewed at frequent intervals. Similar striae and white patches may appear on the vulva and have even been described on the rectal mucosa. Lesions on the glans penis may be papular or annular and if they occur in the absence of lesions elsewhere the patient may develop fear of venereal infection.

A rare variant known as lichen planopilaris may produce irregular scarred patches of permanent alopecia in the scalp and follicular hyperkeratosis over the upper back which gives it the feel of a nutmeg grater.

Children are rarely affected and when they are the lesions are atypical, sometimes giving rise to widespread small verrucose lesions which may be mistaken for psoriasis. Rarely the nails may be involved, usually giving rise to longitudinal ridging and splitting of the nail plate but sometimes causing such severe atrophy of the plate that it is almost completely destroyed. Like psoriasis linear lesions may be produced on the trunk or a limb, having a distribution which falsely suggests neurogenesis. Koebner's phenomenon may also cause lichen planus to become superimposed on other skin lesions, so that as an eczema or exfoliative dermatitis fades and heals, lichen planus may suddenly break out on the same areas.

Aetiology

The aetiology of lichen planus is unknown. It has been thought to be psychogenic and, in a few cases, the coincidence with shock or worry is very striking but the majority of patients can blame nothing specific. Several unrelated drugs can cause an eruption which is identical even to the presence of mouth lesions. Organic arsenicals, gold, mepacrine, chloroquine amiphenazole (Daptazole) and paraminosalicyclic acid (P.A.S.) characteristically cause a lichenoid eruption which in the case of slowly excreted, heavy metals and anti-malarial drugs persists for long after administration has been stopped.

The course of lichen planus is very variable and in general the acute generalised attack seems to resolve more rapidly, the lesions becoming flat, losing their bright colour and turning brown; pigment only may remain after about 3 months. The average duration of the ordinary pattern of lesions is about 6 months. One tenth of patients suffer chronic lesions which last for years, hypertrophic and annular lesions being those which persist the longest. Most patients have only one attack but some suffer recurrences at intervals over many years.

Treatment. There is no specific treatment but in most cases resolution can be speeded by the application of betamethasone valerate or fluocinolone acetonide ointments at night under polythene occlusion. In cases with localised lesions such treatment presents no difficulty but even when lesions are widespread it is possible to treat the arms for a fortnight, then legs, then trunk and if the local application is contained without occlusion on these areas there is usually no recurrence.

Chronic hypertrophic lesions which do not respond to local steroid therapy can be treated by infiltrating the lesion with hydrocortisone or triamcinolone which is injected subcutaneously fortnightly, using 1 ml. per injection.

Ordinary mouth lesions are usually symptomless and require no treatment since they fade with the skin lesions. Ulcerated lesions and those occurring in the absence of skin lesions usually respond to the application of triamcinolone in Orabase twice daily.

When very widespread, the itching can be most distressing and it is helpful to rest the patient in bed while treating with local corticosteroids under polythene occulsion. If there is no response and provided there is no systemic contraindication prednisolone should be given by mouth starting with a dose of 30 mg. daily, maintaining this for 10 to 14 days, in which time eruption should have faded, then gradually weaning the patient off the drug.

CHAPTER 16

DISORDERS OF CIRCULATION

Varicose or gravitational disorders

The largest group of patients with skin lesions of the legs suffer from disorders of venous drainage. The venous circulation of the legs has been likened to a pump which will work satisfactorily only if the valves in the deep veins and the communicating veins between the deep and superficial plexuses are intact, and the muscles of the leg active. Failure of any part of the pump leads to venous insufficiency which results in increased pressure in the venules particularly on walking and standing. This rise in pressure causes hypertrophy of the capillary walls which in turn interferes with the passage of metabolites and blood gases.

Venous insufficiency is caused by:

(i) Obstruction of the deep veins by phlebothrombosis.
(ii) Valvular incompetence after phlebothrombosis.
(iii) Primary valvular incompetence due to congenital absence of valves. (This condition is often hereditary and is associated with varicose veins.)

By far the commonest cause is the post-thrombotic state after child-birth, the patient usually is a middle-aged woman who has had several children and who is overweight. Thrombosis in the deep veins also follows surgical operations, injury to the leg and prolonged bed rest.

Since the deep veins may be grossly damaged without the formation of varicose veins it is incorrect to attribute the complications of venous insufficiency to varicose veins alone and a preferable and more correct name for the condition is gravitational or stasis syndrome.

The complications of venous insufficiency are:

(i) *Pigmentation.* This occurs along the line of varicose veins and around the ankles. Raised capillary pressure forces red cells into the surrounding tissue where the haemoglobin is turned into haemosiderin. Melanin pigmentation may occur where there has been erythema from thrombophlebitis or eczema.

(ii) *Eczema.* Often eczema starts in an area of pigmentation. Erythema and scaling appear and may remain localised and persistent for years. Sudden exacerbation of the eczematous area is often accompanied by a generalised eczematous eruption on the face and forearms. Though infection and local applications may precipitate such a phase some form of auto allergy may be the correct explanation for the onset of gravitational eczema.

(iii) *Atrophie blanche*. White scars often linked together in a network occur on the ankles in patients with venous insufficiency. They resemble scars left by ulceration but are a result of slow necrosis. They occur frequently with blockage of the iliac veins or inferior vena cava.

(iv) *Oedema*. When standing, the normal individual is always on the verge of oedema of the legs. Any rise in venous pressure will cause increased filtration through capillary walls and increase of tissue fluids. In the early stages this may be unnoticed as it collects around the tendo Achilles. Organisation of oedema gives rise to induration and fibrosis which fixes the joints. This limits movement of muscles and adds to the failure of the muscle pump.

Ulceration. A leg suffering from venous insufficiency is liable to ulceration. This occurs usually after a minor injury, such as an abrasion or a bruise which precipitates necrosis of the skin and subcutis. The diagnosis is usually simple since pigmentation, varicosities, induration and oedema are likely to suggest the gravitational origin.

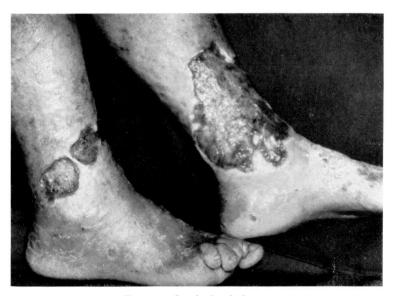

FIG. 75.—Gravitational ulcers.

Avascular ulcers due to arterial insufficiency can be distinguished by a history of claudication and absence of pulsation in peripheral arteries. Essential investigations of any leg ulcer should include a Wassermann reaction, urine examination to exclude diabetes and blood pressure estimation since leg ulcers may occur as a complication of hypertension. A high proportion of patients with chronic leg ulcers develop an iron deficiency anaemia which adds to the tissue malnutrition. In the absence of evidence of venous insufficiency other less common causes of leg ulcers such as blood dyscrasias, rheumatoid arthritis or scleroderma should be sought.

Treatment of gravitational eczema and ulcer

Control of venous hypertension and the removal of oedema by restoration of the venous pump is the primary aim.

An elastic pressure bandage should be applied daily from toes to knee before the patient arises from bed. The bandage should enclose the whole ankle including the heel. If oedema is persistent around the tendo-achilles massage and extra padding with polythene foam Bisgaard treatment (see appendix) may be necessary. If there is gross oedema oral diuretics may also be useful. With the bandage on, walking should be encouraged as walking is good for legs, it is standing which is harmful. The movement of the muscles beneath the elastic support massages fluid up the leg and the increased arterial blood flow and movement of the ankle joint previously fixed by pain and disuse are all beneficial. We see many patients in whom crepe bandages have been prescribed but these do not give sufficient support and are valueless. Elastic stockings are also less effective than elastic bandages and should be reserved for maintenance of support when the ulcer or eczema has healed. Almost as important as firm elastic pressure is weight reduction in the obese and, though frequently difficult to achieve, its value should be impressed on the patient. Many of the elderly are deficient in protein, iron, ascorbic acid and folate and correction of these factors will accelerate recovery.

Local applications to gravitational eczema

In principle, local treatment is the same as it is to eczematous eruptions elsewhere but even more care than usual should be taken to avoid sensitisation to medicaments. Zinc paste B.N.F. as a simple protective with the addition of coal tar 1% if itching is not rapidly relieved is all that is necessary in the mild case. The paste should be covered with Tubegauze and an elastic bandage applied over this. If skin damage by scratching is a marked feature an occlusive bandage of ichthammol or coal tar left in position for a week gives good results. Acute exudative eruptions are an indication for topical steroid lotion or ointment without added antibiotic or antiseptic. If the eczema on the primary site can be controlled quickly the risk of generalised spread of the eruption is reduced. Where possible the patient should remain ambulant and only if severe weeping of the skin and gross oedema of the leg are not controllable then bed rest becomes necessary. Exercises in bed to prevent further phlebothrombosis should be carried out.

Local treatment of leg ulcers

Wet dressings of $\frac{1}{4}$ strength sodium hypochlorite solution are as effective as any other local application and the risk of contact sensitivity is minimal. If steroid applications are used for the treatment of surrounding eczema, care should be taken to prevent any entering the ulcer cavity. Steroids cause vaso-constriction and delay healing. Epithelialisation will not start while sloughs remain in an ulcer. The clearance of sloughs may be hastened by the use of a malic acid preparation Aserbine cream, applied twice daily to the ulcer. We have found a layer of zinc paste applied around the ulcer necessary to prevent irritation of the adjacent skin. When there is a clean granulating surface non adherent rayon squares, Johnsons NA or a proprietary honey and cod liver oil tulle (M and M tulle, Malam Laboratories, Manchester) can be left in position for 3 days at a time. It is a mistake to disturb the epithelialising ulcer more frequently. The healing time of extensive granulating areas can be shortened by the use of multiple small skin grafts applied under paraffin gauze and left in position for 10 days. This simple procedure, using the thigh as a donor area and carried out under local anaesthesia, is safe and effective. Severely infected ulcers should be treated by systemic antibiotics though the exception is when the infecting organism is Bacillus pyocyaneus which can be controlled by gentamycin ointment.

Whatever local treatment is used elastic bandages are essential. In the few patients who will not cooperate an adhesive elastic bandage (Elastoplast) can be substituted. Skin irritation can be avoided by applying a calamine impregnated bandage beneath or applying adhesive bandage with the resin surface outwards. When the ulcer has healed the majority of patients still need elastic support, possibly only elastic stockings, and weight reduction must be maintained. To avoid recurrent ulceration surgical treatment, either by ligation or injection of perforating veins around the malleoli or the stripping of varicose veins must be considered but careful investigation and possible venography are advisable before surgery is embarked upon.

Arterial ulcers

Necrosis of the skin of the leg from anoxia occurs in patients with peripheral arterial disease, frequently a complication of diabetes. There is usually a history of claudication in the calf muscles. The ulcers which are usually higher up the leg than venous ulcers are covered by a dry, hard slough. The skin of the foot is shiny, the toes are likely to be cold and blue or with a dull erythema and no pulsation can be felt in the peripheral vessels.

Treatment. It is important to recognise the arterial insufficiency as elastic bandages are contra-indicated. Exercises, control of diabetes if present, systemic antibiotics and bed rest may permit slow healing to take place. Eventually amputation of the limb may be necessary if reconstructive arterial surgery is not possible.

There is considerable individual variation in the vascular supply of the skin of the face and limbs and in particular its response to heat and cold.

Livedo reticularis (Marbled skin)

This is an exaggeration of the normal vascular pattern seen on the limbs in children and young adults. Islands of white skin are surrounded by a bluish, pink network where the blood flow is more sluggish. This network of vessels can be made permanently visible by prolonged exposure to heat from the fire or hot water bottle which gives rise to erythema and pigmentation (erythema ab igne). After puberty many girls develop cold blue swelling of the lower third of the legs (erythrocyanosis crurum) associated with a liability to chilblains. A similar bluish response of the hands and feet to cold is termed acrocyanosis.

Chilblains

Chilblains are caused by exposure of susceptible individuals to cold; not only must the extremities be cooled but chilling of the whole body is an important factor. Chilblains are dusky red, itchy swellings which occur mainly on the fingers and toes but can extend up the backs of the legs and occasionally occur on areas such as the buttocks, the nose and ears. The swelling and burning are a result of the active hyperaemia which follows a period of spasm of the small arterioles induced by cold.

Treatment. The best simple preventive measures are designed to prevent body chilling. Sedentary workers in cold surroundings are more liable to suffer from chilblains than active, out-of-door workers exposed to much lower temperatures. Adequate heating of offices, shops and schools, physical exercise and the wearing of warm clothing are of more value than drugs. Exposure of the chilblain areas to intensive ultraviolet light just before the winter has been shown to prevent chilblains by increasing the skin blood flow for some months, but we have found this an unreliable method of treatment. When chilblains have developed inunction of the following gives symptomatic relief, Balsam of Peru and camphor 3% of each in lanolin and soft paraffin equal parts. Calcium and calciferol which have long been used are ineffective but some relief may be obtained by the use of vasodilator drugs such as nicotinic acid 100 mg. or dibenyline (Phenoxybenzamine) 10 mg. twice daily.

Raynaud's phenomenon

A more serious reaction to cold is that of Raynaud's phenomenon. The manifestations are due to arteriolar vasoconstriction of the vessels

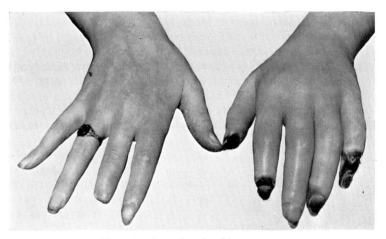

FIG. 76.—Acrosclerosis with gangrene.

of the fingers and, less commonly, the toes, nose and ears. The fingers become cold, dead white for a period of several minutes to several hours. When the spasm of the vessel diminishes, the fingers become blue, hot and painful. Whilst this response to cold may persist with little structural change for many years, in some patients the symptoms denote the onset of a chronic systemic disease, systemic sclerosis or scleroderma, now recognised as one of the auto-immune diseases. The condition, which is more common in women than in men, involves the connective tissue of the whole body and severe irreversible changes take place in the dermis, kidney, lung, heart and gastro-intestinal tract. After the initial Raynaud's phenomenon the fingers become stiffened with binding down of the dermis to the deeper tissues and gradual tapering and atrophy of the finger tips which is called acrosclerosis. This stage may last many years before systemic organs appear to be involved. The face and mouth are frequently affected and this gives rise to a characteristic facies with a shrunken mouth and beak nose. Telangiectases appear also on the face and hands. Dysphagia is complained of when the oesophagus is involved, though X-ray

6

changes may be found even without symptoms. The course is progressively downhill with acute episodes of gangrene of the extremities
associated with ulceration and calcification. No curative treatment
exists for systemic sclerosis but sympathectomy is of some value in
Raynaud's disease not associated with scleroderma.

Localised scleroderma or morphoea

This is histologically due to a similar change in the dermal collagen
to the systemic disease but is a harmless disorder. Circumscribed
patches of hardened ivory coloured skin with a violaceous border
appear usually on the trunk though occasionally a segmental or nerve
distribution is seen. Local injection of steroids or the application of
steroid ointment under polythene have been used but give disappoint-
ingly poor results but spontaneous resolution occurs in a considerable
number of patients. Closely allied to localised scleroderma is another
disorder known as lichen sclerosus et atrophicus. This differs only in
that the lesions are usually smaller and there is frequent involvement
of the vulva in women.

Bedsores

Pressure sores develop in bedridden patients if they are left lying
inert bearing their weight for hours on the same bony areas. Thus a
patient lying on his back develops pressure sores over the sacrum, the
backs of the heels and the scapulae. Constant pressure on these points
impairs the blood supply to the skin and subcutaneous tissues so that
they develop a localised gangrene. If the patient is in a state of collapse,
so that the normal blood supply to the skin is already reduced, such
lesions can form very rapidly; for example someone who collapses
unattended at home and lies unconscious on a hard floor for about
12 hours before being found, may already be developing sores on
the points of pressure.

Maceration of the skin in the incontinent patient makes the development of bedsores more probable. In those skin diseases such as pemphigus in which large areas of skin become eroded as part of the disease
process, bedsores are extremely difficult to prevent.

Once formed, bedsores are very difficult to heal and every possible
preventive measure should be adopted from the start of the patient's
illness. In a very ill patient who is needing a lot of attention and may
have to be somewhat immobilised for transfusion of fluids it is only
too easy to give insufficient attention to the pressure areas until it is
too late. The patient should be moved or encouraged to move, or to
lie for 2 hours on one side then for 2 hours on the other. If the patient's
general condition allows, even though the skin may be severely diseased,
he should be got out of bed and sat in a chair for an hour or two each

day to take pressure off the heels and sacrum. The very ill patient who cannot be got out of bed can be nursed on a ripple mattress which by varied inflation alters the points bearing weight. Possibly even better than the ripple mattress is a sheepskin of which a special type which is very easy to clean is available. When the patient has to sit up, an inflatable air ring takes pressure off the sacrum but sometimes defeats its object by making it difficult for the patient to move himself. Also in the sitting patient padded rings should be bound on the heels to lift them off the bed or an oblong block of foam rubber or polythene 4–6 inches thick can be cut to extend from the knee to the ankle and placed under calves so that the heels are elevated off the bed.

The traditional practice of rubbing the back with spirit—which is in any case of doubtful value—is out of the question in cases of generalised skin disease. Talc powder dusted over the back and into the underlying areas of the bed absorbs sweat and reduces friction. The incontinent patient presents an additional difficulty and obviously the draw sheet should be changed whenever soiled so that the skin does not become macerated. The application of an oily cream B.P. to the back and buttocks twice daily also helps to waterproof the skin and prevent maceration. If these precautions are meticulously observed pressure sores should not develop.

Unfortunately occasionally patients have already developed pressure scores at home before they come under nursing care. In such cases the first line of treatment is removal of pressure from the sore by the methods already detailed.

The multitude of ideas on what is the best application for the established pressure sore indicates that none is of outstanding value and suggests that most are virtually useless. We have found cod-liver oil and honey tulle (M & M tulle) to be a safe, comfortable and satisfactory application. If the ulcer is deep it can be packed with the tulle; if shallow applied once daily. The healing of any ulcer depends at least as much on the patient's general condition as on local applications. Large bedsores produce toxaemia which can lead to death and always depress blood formation causing anaemia. Improvement in the underlying disease, correction of anaemia with blood transfusion if necessary, maintenance of an adequate diet and vitamin supplements are all valuable moves in the battle against an established bedsore.

CHAPTER 17

DISORDERS OF SEBACEOUS AND SWEAT GLANDS

Sebaceous glands are formed as a diverticulum of the epithelial lining of the hair follicle into which they open towards the surface of the skin. They are composed of solid lobulated masses of cells which, from the periphery to the centre, become progressively filled with fat granules. The glands are of the type in which secretion entails disintegration of the cells, the resultant mixture of cellular debris and fatty matter forming sebum. The only areas free from sebaceous glands are the palms and soles and areas of most profuse secretion are the nose, forehead and central chest, the amount secreted diminishing to the sides of the chest and back.

Increased sebaceous gland activity commences at puberty and has been shown to be influenced by an increase in androgens secreted by adrenals and gonads. The final stage of steroid metabolism, probably converting precursors to active androgens or even testosterone itself, takes place in the sebaceous gland cells and there is an increased steroid metabolic turnover in the areas of most profuse secretion. About the age of 25 years adult levels of secretion are reached and remain static.

Acne vulgaris

Acne vulgaris commences at puberty and results from this overactivity of the sebaceous glands, its distribution on the face, central chest and back corresponding to areas of highest secretion of sebum. The sex incidence is equal, so that the amount of androgen secreted must matter less than the sensitivity of the sebaceous glands to its presence. This appears to be an hereditary sensitivity, but it is still not clear why some children develop increased sebaceous activity with only occasional and scanty acne lesions, while in others sebaceous flow is blocked by thickening of the horny layer at the opening of the hair follicles, especially the lanugo hairs on the face, damming up the sebum and leading to profuse acne lesions.

Hyperkeratosis and inspissation of sebum in the follicle produces the comedo or blackhead which is the primary lesion of acne vulgaris. The resultant blockage of the gland and statis of the contents enables the resident saprophytic organisms (Pityrosporon ovale, Corynebacterium acnes and coagulase negative staphylococci) to break down the lipids in sebum and produce free fatty acids which leak into the dermis,

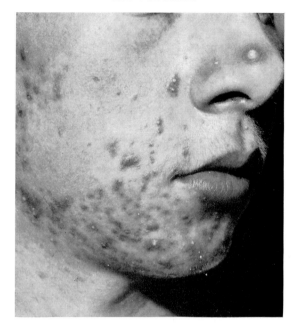

FIG. 77.—Acne vulgaris.

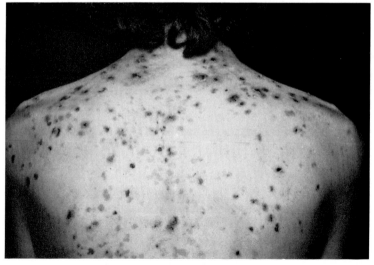

FIG. 78.—Acne vulgaris.

causing an inflammatory reaction and the formation of a red papule. This inflammatory response may produce pus which points onto the surface as a pustule. Since the pus formation results from a foreign body reaction rather than infection these pustules are usually sterile or contain saprophytic organisms. A greater degree of reaction may not point to the surface but may remain dammed up in the corium to form a cyst.

The full picture of acne consists then of comedones, papules and pustules on face, neck, back, chest and sometimes upper arms; in severe cases these lesions are accompanied by cysts.

Once established other factors have some influence over the course of acne. There is no evidence that sebaceous glands are under nervous control but there is no doubt that mental stress can aggravate acne; as an example lesions may become much worse in adolescents working for examinations. The severity of acne in adolescents with epilepsy is also notable. In girls there is usually a premenstrual exacerbation of lesions.

Diet is not likely to affect acne vulgaris appreciably but consumption of chocolate and cocoa can aggravate the lesions. Iodides and bromides not only cause an acneiform eruption as a toxic side effect but also aggravate existing acne.

Climatic factors also influence the course and extent of the lesions; exposure to sun and wind, increasing desquamation of the exposed skin diminishes the hyperkeratosis of the hair follicles and reduces comedone formation. Acne can therefore be shown to be more common and severe in the smoke screened North of England than in the relatively sunny South.

Its severity diminishes in the late teens and in the majority of patients lesions cease to appear in the early twenties. Rarely lesions persist into older age groups in those suffering from a rare familial form and in those in whom acne progresses to acne rosacea. In men acne is particularly liable to persist over the back until middle age. In women acne papules may recur on the chin in the premenstrual phase for many years and sometimes recur throughout the reproductive period of life.

Treatment should be aimed at tiding the patient over the acne years with as few lesions as possible to diminish the psychological trauma of a spotty face and the appearance of scarring, which if severe may produce disfigurement for life.

Dietary restrictions have so little effect that the only one worth imposing is on chocolate. Exposure to fresh air and sunshine is advice not easy to follow but it helps by increasing desquamation. Other treatment is aimed at degreasing and desquamating the skin, suppressing sebaceous glandular activity and suppressing inflammatory reaction.

Detergents should be prescribed to degrease the skin and used for cleaning the face instead of soap and water. Cetrimide (Cetavlon) in 1% solution or proprietary detergent bars are suitable.

Sulphur applications induce desquamation; sulphurated potash lotion is relatively mild and should be applied twice daily by dabbing on with cotton wool or the finger tips. If this fails to produce desquamation the stronger application of Lassar's paste with 3% sulphur and resorcin may be applied at night only; this is rather difficult to remove and Brasivol ointment in its increasing strengths may be more acceptable to the patient. In girls a cosmetic to hide the lesions may be combined with sulphur and resorcin and is available in several proprietary applications. Sulphur may also be added to a cosmetic-type base such as Collosol Calamine (Crooke's) with 1–2% precipitated sulphur. The patient should be discouraged from squeezing out comedones with finger nails or comedone expressors as scarring may result. Local corticosteroids have little beneficial effect on acne and the stronger ones are particularly undesirable as they eventually produce a scaly telangiectatic erythema of the muzzle area which has been termed perioral dermatitis.

If local applications are insufficient, desquamation may be produced by erythema doses of ultraviolet light 2 or 3 times weekly, but usually improvement is only maintained during the course of treatment. Prolonged administration of a small dose of oxytetracycline effectively suppresses the inflammatory lesions in most cases. Treatment should commence with 250 mg. twice daily until the lesions are controlled, which usually takes 4 to 6 weeks, then the dose is reduced to 250 mg. daily for weeks or months to maintain control. During its administration there is a reduction in free fatty acids in the sebum which could be due to the bacteriostatic effect of tetracycline on the fat splitting saprophytic organisms. However this is unlikely to be the whole explanation as in some cases the relapse on stopping tetracycline is dramatic in its speed and severity.

After trying these measures without success it is justifiable to arrange X-ray therapy, which acts by suppressing the activity of sebaceous glands over a period of about 9 months. The usual course is 100 rads at 40 kV on three occasions at intervals of 2 weeks and improvement is to be expected about a month after the last dose. If a relapse occurs, the same course may be repeated after a year but it is important to bear in mind that no single area of skin should receive more than 1000 rads in a lifetime.

Oestrogens administered systemically suppress sebaceous activity and improve acne. Since the availability of tetracycline they are hardly ever necessary or justifiable in the male. In the female the contraceptive pill with a high oestrogen content benefited some cases without upsetting the menstrual cycle. The present low oestrogen pill is less effective.

When uncontrolled acne has been severe the degree of scarring which remains may be very disfiguring. A period of at least a year after the acne lesions have ceased should allow some resolution of the scars and, if still marked, planing of the face by dermabrasion can produce considerable improvement.

Acne rosacea

The lesions of acne rosacea are usually confined to the flush areas of the forehead, nose, cheeks and chin and result from over-activity of the sebaceous glands induced by hyperaemia. Rarely lesions may appear on the neck, the V-area of the chest and the upper arms. Unlike acne vulgaris there is no blockage of the ducts and therefore comedones are

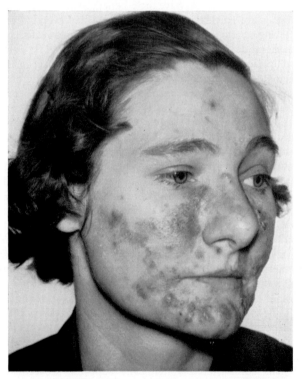

FIG. 79.—Rosacea.

not formed but inflammation occurs round the hypertrophied glands producing papules and pustules or rarely cysts. Like acne vulgaris these pustules are sterile or contain saprophytes.

Since facial flushing is the initial lesion acne rosacea may be caused by any of the reasons for chronic flush. Usually the subjects have shown lifelong evidence of vasomotor instability which is in many cases familial. In such subjects psychological stress—said by the psychiatrists to be feelings of guilt, social insecurity or suppressed rage—can lead to a chronic flush and resultant acne lesions. There are certain groups of rosacea patients in whom local factors appear more potent than the psyche; in the late twenties and thirties, what was acne vulgaris may persist as acne rosacea with continuing over-activity of the sebaceous glands; in women suffering from menopausal flushes, endocrine factors are important; in both sexes, but more often in the male, chronic alcoholism produces a persistent flush. However, when subjected to statistical analysis the relevance of these factors is submerged in the large group of patients from whom no such explanation can be elicited.

Hypertrophy of the sebaceous glands may occur to such a degree on the nose that it becomes bulbous and lobulated, a condition known as rhinophyma. A more serious complication is involvement of the eye. Many sufferers from acne rosacea show symptoms of the seborrhoeic diathesis, such as scurfy scalp and blepharitis. With attacks of blepharitis they may also develop conjunctivitis. A less easily understood complication is keratitis. This may recur at times when rosacea is little evident and is prone to remissions and recurrences. It may lead to a severe vascularising superficial keratitis, usually bilateral, giving rise to photophobia, lacrimation and visual failure. Corneal lesions develop as patches of opacity spreading in from the corneal margin.

Treatment. The patient must be advised to avoid those things which may produce flushing of the face such as sitting over a hot fire, drinking hot drinks, especially of tea, and taking too hot or spiced foods. Alcohol should be forbidden or taken only with meals. Where mental stress is caused by alterable circumstance, help and advice may benefit the patient, but psychiatric treatment on grounds of the psychosomatic nature of the skin disease is doomed to failure.

Locally sulphur lotions are helpful and as some form of covering lotion is a help psychologically an elegant cosmetic preparation can be made by adding 2% precipitated sulphur to Collosol Calamine lotion. In some cases, associated seborrhoeic dermatitis causes an additional scaly erythema and here 2% precipitated sulphur and salicyclic acid, in aqueous cream is helpful. The potent corticosteroid applications should never be used as they produce atrophy of the facial skin and increase telangiectasia; but hydrocortisone, either as the cream or combined with sulphur in a proprietary preparation is beneficial in some cases and apparently harmless.

The administration of a low dose of oxytetracycline over a prolonged period is even more successful in acne rosacea than in acne vulgaris. Treatment should commence with 250 mg. of tetracycline twice daily until the eruption is controlled and the dose then reduced to 250 mg. Such maintenance treatment can be stopped after a month in many cases, but some may need continuous treatment for many months. Such antibiotic therapy also suppresses blepharitis and may have some effect on keratitis.

Acne rosacea fluctuates in severity from day to day and from year to year. It may undergo long periods of remission which probably depend upon the patient's mental welfare but once established recurrences are common and the routine of treatment must be devised with this in mind so that radiotherapy should be a last resort. When it is used the dosage is similar to that prescribed for acne vulgaris (q.v.).

Local applications have no influence on rhinophyma but a good cosmetic result can be achieved by the simple operation of paring off the excess tissue of the nose and leaving it to re-epithelialise, which it does rapidly as the remnants of hypertrophied sebaceous glands act as scattered seeds of epithelium.

Acne necrotica

Acne necrotica is an uncommon chronic folliculitis which characteristically affects the hair margin of the forehead and temples, though it may extend into the scalp. Staphylococcal infection is responsible for the lesions but nearly always the patients are suffering from psychological stress or an anxiety state, the lesions are irritable and the habit of picking at them aggravates the condition. Acneiform papules are produced with a small necrotic crust at the centre which heal leaving a varioliform scar. The lesions heal rapidly on treatment with oxytetracycline 250 mg. twice daily; mild cases may simply require local antibiotic therapy. A maintenance dose of oxytetracycline is often required and treatment of the mental state when this is appropriate.

Disorders of sweating

Sweat glands are formed in embryo life as off-shoots of epidermal cells. They number 100–200 glands per sq. cm. and are even greater in number on the forehead, palms and soles. Their function is to flood the skin surface with water for cooling and the prime stimulus to activity is heat. Thermoregulation is a function of the hypothalamus and an increase in skin temperature or in blood temperature results in hypothalamic discharges which are carried to the sweat glands by the sympathetic nervous system. There is no inhibitory innervation of the glands and resection of sympathetic fibres results in anhidrosis.

Apart from the stimulus of heat the sweat glands are influenced reflexly by stimuli such as the sight of heat; also by the emotional stresses of pain, fear or anger which especially provoke sweating on the palms, soles, axillae and forehead.

Anhidrosis may occur as a generalised or localised phenomenon resulting from damage to the hypothalamus or interference with the sympathetic supply to the sweat glands. More important is the generalised anhidrosis which occurs from lack of function or congenital absence of sweat glands and which is most easily recognised in ichthyosis. Because of their inability to regulate heat loss such subjects are prone to heat stroke and should avoid tropic or sub-tropic climates.

Localised hyperhidrosis is usually produced by emotional tension and is commonly complained of when it affects the palms or axillae. Advice concerning the cause of the stress should help, occasionally the aid of a psychiatrist is necessary. Sedation with chlordiazepoxide 10 mg. thrice daily and the application of 10% sodium hetametaphosphate solution to the areas of sweating several times daily usually controls the symptom. Sympathetic inhibitory drugs are ineffective in our experience. When axillary sweating is the only complaint excision of an elipse of skin from the apex of the axillae reduces sweating but in many cases the improvement is transient. Rarely palmar sweating may be severe enough to interfere with the patient's work and in such cases cervical sympathectomy is successful.

Hyperhidrosis of the soles and its unpleasant odour are more common complaints not often traceable to an emotional cause. The skin of the soles becomes red, tender and macerated; the macerated skin has a "worm eaten" appearance and as thick white soggy skin also appears between the toes it is sometimes mistaken for tinea pedis. The patient should avoid rubber soled shoes and should wear sandals when possible in hot weather. Soaking the soles in 3% formalin solution for 5 to 10 minutes each night or the application of 10% glutaraldehyde solution on a cottonwool swab 3 times a week are both very effective.

Miliaria rubra or prickly heat is the bane of the tropics to white races. The eruption occurs in humid hot weather as sheets of erythematous papulo-vesicles on the trunk, especially round the waist and on the antecubital and popliteal fossae. Intensely itchy, the lesions fluctuate from day to day according to the temperature. The mechanism is formation of a keratin plug in the sweat duct as the result of maceration of the skin. When sweating occurs, the occluded duct ruptures into the epidermis and escaping sweat forms an intra-epidermal-vesicle. Invasion by staphylococci probably plays a secondary role.

Treatment consists of reduction of sweating produced by exertion or excessive clothing, promotion of evaporation from the skin surface and thus cooling by the use of fans or, ideally, air conditioning. Topically neomycin lotion gives some relief by reducing bacterial invasion; ascorbic acid 1000 mg. daily has been shown to be effective in the Far East.

The papulo-pustular eruption often seen on the face and sometimes the trunk of babies in the first few weeks of life probably has a similar mode of production, though here excessive clothing and high nursery temperature are the cause. It too responds quickly to lowering of the temperature.

CHAPTER 18

DISORDERS OF PIGMENTATION

NORMAL pigmentation of the skin is due to melanin, whose role is that of a light barrier. It is synthesised by melanocytes which are distributed among the basal cells of the epidermis and in the hair matrix. These melanocytes are embryologically derived from the neural crest and they inject melanin into the epidermal cells through dendritic processes. The depth of colour of the skin is genetically determined, yet the number of melanocytes in white or negro skin is the same, the difference in pigmentation resulting from greater activity of the melanocytes. Albinism is a recessive congenital defect in the melanocytes leading to failure of pigment formation.

The melanocytes are under the control of a melanocyte stimulating hormone of the anterior pituitary (M.S.H.). Increased production of this hormone occurs in pregnancy and causes darkening of the nipples, genitalia and linea alba, also chloasma a patchy pigmentation of the face especially marked on the temples which is a common side effect of the contraceptive pill. Production of M.S.H. is probably regulated by other hormones, in particular by hydrocortisone, so that damage to the adrenals by Addison's disease leads to release of M.S.H. and causes generalised pigmentation, most marked on the axillae, nipples, genitalia and also present on the buccal mucosa. Similarly increased production of M.S.H. may cause pigmentation in hyperthyroidism and chronic liver disease. Decreased pigmentation results from damage to the pituitary in hypopituitarism and acromegaly and is also seen in eunuchs.

Melanin is derived from tyrosine which is manufactured in the body from the essential amino-acid phenylalanine. Tyrosine is first converted to dihydroxyphenylalanine (D.O.P.A.) which is then converted to dopaquinone then melanin. The stage of conversion of tyrosine to D.O.P.A. is dependent on the copper containing enzyme tyrosinase and in this reaction dopa itself acts as a catalyst. The enzyme tyrosinase is inhibited by a compound containing sulphydryl groups.

Interference with this chain of melanogenesis can produce disorders of pigmentation. At its basic step a high blood level of phenylalanine can lead to competitive inhibition of the enzyme tyrosinase; such a metabolic defect occurs in the inherited disorder of phenylketonuria and results in hypopigmentation of the hair and skin. Elimination of phenylalanine from the diet or oral administration of tyrosine partially restores colour to the hair. Tyrosinase is also inhibited by an antioxidant placed in rubber (monobenzyl ether of hydroquinone) as the result of which the wearing of rubber gloves has caused depigmentation of the hands in negroes.

Inorganic arsenic inactivates the sulphydryl groups in the tyrosinase inhibitor, freeing tyrosinase and causing pigmentation of the skin. Sunlight is also thought to inhibit the sulphydryl compound, releasing tyrosinase to cause a rapid localised increase in melanogenesis. The effects of sunlight are increased by photosensitisers of which industrial exposure to tar provides the most striking picture of pigmentation on the light-exposed areas. A similar industrial pigmentation is sometimes produced by mineral oils used as coolants in engineering.

Increase in pigmentation commonly follows inflammation of the skin and here again the mechanism is thought to be inactivation of the sulphydryl groups. Such pigmentation is particularly marked after lichen planus.

In conditions in which the epidermal cells are proliferating rapidly, such as psoriasis, there is a failure in the transport of melanin granules causing depigmentation in healed areas. Similar depigmentation occurs after eczema in the Negro. Increase in the horny layer may also screen the skin from the tanning effects of ultraviolet light, producing depigmented macules in tinea versicolor and also in the mild patchy scaly dermatitis which may be produced on the faces of children by the effects of strong soap or cold winds. The latter condition heals with the avoidance of soap and the application of hydrocortisone or lanoline ointment.

Partial depigmentation occurs in the macular lesions of leprosy (q.v.).

Melanoderma

Patchy pigmentation of the face is occasionally complained of by women and may produce different patterns affecting the forehead and cheeks or mainly the peribuccal area. Reticulate patterns can be formed by the pigment and sometimes it is accompanied by telangiectasia. In such cases light sensitisation has usually been provoked by oil of bergamot which contains as the sensitising agent 5-methoxypsoralen. Oil of bergamot is widely used in the perfume industry and has commonly been applied in a face cream. More obvious pigmentation provoked by this perfume can be seen when scent runs down the side of the neck and produces a pigment streak.

Treatment. Such patients should be advised to stop using all perfumed cosmetics and avoid exposure to sunlight. It may take many months for the pigmentation to fade. The inhibiting effect on melanin formation of hydroquinone has been used to hasten the paling of such areas of pigmentation. It is applied in 2% concentration in a cream base, but is liable to produce dermatitis.

Vitiligo is a condition of unknown aetiology which affects about

1 per cent of the population. Depigmented patches appear in the skin, which retains its normal texture. The failure of melanogenesis which occurs in these areas is thought to be due to a reduction in the number or complete absence of normal melanocytes.

Vitiligo may begin at any age but more commonly before the age of 20. About half the subjects can trace it in another member of their family and it is seen in association with the organ specific autoimmune diseases of the thyroid, pernicious anaemia, diabetes mellitus and also alopecia areata in a significant number of cases. In a few patients the onset is associated with physical or mental stress. The disorder has periods of quiescence and progression that are unpredictable and ultimately large areas of the skin can be affected, yet in about 50 per cent of patients some repigmentation occurs.

Treatment. The only treatment which has any effect is the use of oral psoralen compounds. 8-Methoxypsoralen (Methoxsalen) has been given in a dose of 10-20 mg. twice daily and also applied locally. In countries where natural sunlight is a reliable commodity the patient is exposed to an increasing dose about 2 hours after a tablet and good results are reported. The use of other sources of U.V.L. such as the cold quartz lamp or "Blacklite" give disappointing results in our experience. Only about 15 per cent of patients so treated achieve any repigmentation, recently developed patches are more likely to respond and there is a better response on the covered areas of the body and limbs than on the face, which is usually the area causing most concern. Repigmentation can only be maintained by prolonged therapy, disappearing within 2 years when treatment is stopped. Trimethylpsoralen (Trisoralen) gives better results on exposed areas such as hands and face but complete repigmentation only occurs in the minority of cases and increased pigmentation of the normal skin makes the condition even more obtrusive in the rest. In white patients satisfactory cosmetic results can be achieved by advising the patient to avoid exposure to sunshine, which increases pigmentation of the normal skin and by disguising the white patches with a cosmetic covering cream or dihydroxyacetone paint.

Non-melanin pigmentation

Argyria due to deposition of silver salts in the skin produces a slate grey pigmentation which is still seen in silversmiths.

Haemochromatosis is a rare disorder of iron metabolism in which diabetes is found. Iron salts and melanin are responsible for the patient's bronze colour.

CHAPTER 19

THE SKIN AND EMOTIONAL DISORDER

ONE cannot treat patients suffering from skin disease without becoming acutely aware that many ascribe correctly aggravation of their
symptoms to emotional tensions. The exact mechanism by which a
condition such as atopic eczema or psoriasis can be influenced by
anxiety is unknown but it is reasonable to suppose that skin blood flow
and the activity of sweat glands may be altered by stress. In the management of chronic skin disorders therefore an awareness that social and
emotional factors are of importance is essential.

Perhaps less often recognised is the effect of skin disorder on the
personality of the sufferer. Many adolescents are disturbed by the
unsightliness of acne vulgaris and what may appear to be a trivial and
commonplace dermatosis can produce very real suffering in the boy or
girl who has to face the world with a pimply face. Itching destroys
morale equally as much as pain and until the advent of the anti-inflammatory steroids little attention was paid to the effect of chronic itching and
sleeplessness on the personality of the sufferer. It is very striking that
sufferers from atopic eczema tend to be aggressive, yet this attitude can
be changed rapidly by relief of their symptoms by systemic steroids.
In addition there are a number of patients who present with symptoms
referable to their skin who are suffering from mental disorder.

Cutaneous hypochondriasis

Some patients become morbidly anxious about what may be a physio-
logical anomaly. The following are examples of this condition; the
patient who notices the circumvallate papillae on the tongue or the
submucous sebaceous glands on the buccal mucosa (Fordyces spots),
which are present in more than 50% of normal individuals. The patient
develops a possible cancer phobia and may be difficult to reassure.
A particularly difficult problem is the patient with syphilophobia who
refuses to be reassured despite numerous negative blood tests. More
bizarre cutaneous delusions may be the first evidence of schizophrenia.
The belief that the patient is being avoided by his friends because of
some trivial blemish or from imagined body odour are common
methods of presentation.

Delusion of parasitosis. Parasitophobia

Some people are convinced that the skin is infested with parasites
and frequently display a collection of skin scales and rolled up keratin

in support of their theory. The patient is usually elderly with an obsessional personality and unfortunately neither dermatological or psychiatric therapy offers much hope.

Dermatitis artefacta

It is difficult to accept the idea that patients can and do inflict lesions on their own skins yet such is the case. Though numerically unimportant, factitious lesions may be so chronic and may have medicolegal implications that some consideration should be given to them.

As a clinical problem dermatitis artefacta should be suspected if superficial ulcerated lesions fail to heal despite prolonged conventional treatment. A clue may be gained from the character of the lesion which may have a bizarre shape (square or rectangular) which does not conform to natural disease. Confirmation of the diagnosis may be obtained by speedy healing of the lesions under occlusive dressings if this is practicable.

The patient should not be questioned directly about the possibility of artefact as the emotional reaction is likely to be violent but the possibility of psychogenic stresses should be investigated.

Young girls frequently produce lesions as a hysterical reaction to draw attention to their problems, whereas in older age groups a true

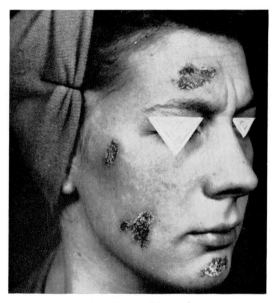

FIG. 80.—Dermatitis artefacta.

psychosis is more likely, though occasionally artefacts are produced for financial gain.

Neurotic excoriations

Patients who are emotionally labile may inflict deep excoriations on the parts of the skin which they can reach easily with their finger nails.

The clinical picture of superficial excoriations scattered on the limbs and shoulders, but sparing the centre of the back, and the presence of numerous white healed scars is characteristic. The skin damage is not a result of deliberate intent as in dermatitis artefacta but due to uncontrollable impulses. Occlusion will allow skin lesions to heal and assist in the confirmation of the diagnosis but the prognosis is not good and psychiatric assistance is usually needed.

Acne excoriée

A variant of neurotic excoriations in the young female adolescent is the picking and squeezing of pustules and comedones of acne vulgaris. Often the scarring of the excoriations far exceeds the severity of the acne. The underlying emotional stresses must be investigated to achieve improvement.

Trichotillomania

Rubbing, twisting and pulling the hair is a common habit in children which causes a thinning of the scalp hair. Examination reveals that the hair shafts are broken and the alopecia is always incomplete with hairs of varying lengths. Treatment consists in the discovery of why the child is tense and explanation to the parents that the habit will cease in time if no attention is paid to it. Rarely, trichotillomania may also occur in adults when it may be superimposed occasionally on alopecia areata or appear as a self-inflicted mutilation.

CHAPTER 20

DISORDERS OF THE HAIR

HAIR is formed from hard keratin by the matrix cells of the hair follicles which are invaginations of the epidermis. The extra-follicular hair is a dead structure and no procedures applied to it will have any stimulating effect on its growth. There are two types of hair, the fine, downy, vellus hair which is present over the whole body except the palms and soles, and terminal hairs, the thick, pigmented hairs which are present on the scalp, beard, eyebrows, eyelashes, axillary, pubic and body regions.

Hair growth occurs in cycles and hair in different regions has a different growth cycle. A long growing phase (anagen) is followed by involution of the follicles and a short resting phase (telogen). Resting hairs make up 5–15 per cent of the total of 100,000 hairs on the human scalp and the daily loss of scalp hair is 20–100. Scalp hair grows about 2 mm. weekly and the growing phase of any one hair is 2 to 3 years, though exceptionally it may be very much longer. Terminal hairs elsewhere on the body have a shorter growing phase than those on the scalp. The high speed of growth of the scalp hair makes it more susceptible to damage from systemic disease, toxic drugs and radiation.

Hair growth is dependent on hormone influences and hair in different regions is dependent on different hormone stimulants. Oestrogens are a stimulant to scalp hair growth in women and androgens have the reverse effect. During pregnancy there is a delay in telogen hair fall so that scalp hair becomes thicker than normal. A sudden hair fall occurs in the puerperium and this is most marked in the frontal areas. Hair is also lost after the menopause and there may be at the same time an increase in facial hair growth. Axillary and pubic hair is dependent in women on adrenal androgens and the hair is lost in Addison's disease, whilst in men the hair is not lost as testosterone alone can maintain it. In contrast, testosterone has a deleterious effect on male scalp hair and eunuchs do not develop male pattern baldness. In hypothyroidism and in hypoparathyroidism, the hair on the scalp and the whole body becomes dry and sparse. Therapeutic corticosteroids behave like androgens and overgrowth of vellus hair is an undesirable side effect.

Alopecia, or hair loss, can occur as a result of changes in the hair follicles which are invisible or from manifest disease of the scalp which destroys the hair matrices. So much psychological significance is attached to the possession of luxuriant scalp hair that a complaint of thinning hair is a frequent one. It is important to assess that the symptoms are real since many women do not appreciate that the loss of 100 hairs a day is normal and as part of an anxiety state believe that they are going bald. The daily hair loss can be checked by asking the patient to collect the hairs removed by a comb and they can then be counted.

Hair loss from systemic disease

Diffuse hair fall some three months after a severe febrile illness is common and it may also occur after extensive surgical procedures. Regrowth of hair is invariable in three to four months. Less commonly, hair fall may occur with severe emotional stress. Hair loss in a patient with rheumatoid arthritis may indicate the onset of disseminated lupus erythematosus and though now rare, syphilis should be excluded in the diagnosis of patchy alopecia. The antimitotic drugs, and heparin and dextran all cause profuse alopecia. A lowered serum iron either due to frequent blood loss from disease or from repeated donation of blood transfusions may cause diffuse hair loss.

Puerperal alopecia

As has already been mentioned, a male pattern of baldness and frontal recession may appear in women about three months after childbirth and this can return more severely in successive pregnancies. Regrowth

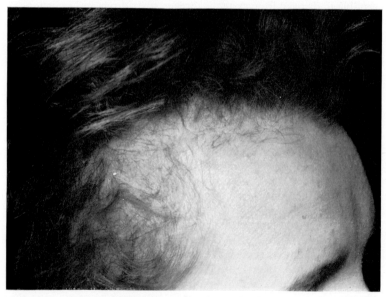

FIG. 81.—Puerperal hair loss.

is already taking place when hair loss is noticed and no treatment other than reassurance is necessary.

Male pattern baldness

Loss of hair on the frontal region and over the vertex may begin soon after puberty in males. Once begun, baldness progresses with phases of active hair loss followed by static periods. Increased dandruff, erythema and irritation occur coincident with the hair fall. This appears to be an associated androgen effect and not the cause of the hair loss. Hair follicles can be transferred by grafting from the occipital to the frontal region and the resultant hairs will continue to grow. This suggests that the growth factor for occipital hair and frontal hairs is different. It is not a practicable treatment for male baldness and prognosis for hair recovery is hopeless. There is, of course, a strong genetic factor in male baldness and patients should be discouraged from seeking a medical cure and advised to accept their fate philosophically.

Hair loss in women

Thinning of the scalp hair over the vertex and top of the head is common in menopausal women and marked baldness may occur in extreme old age. In recent years, more young women have complained of early baldness, which may reflect the general increased interest in hair styling rather than an absolute increase in the condition. Investigation rarely reveals any endocrine disorder although hypothyroidism is responsible for a small number. Excess of virilising hormones is extremely rare but must be excluded. The hair loss is similar to male baldness and like it, has a strong genetic factor. Fortunately, the baldness is only partial and rarely noticeable to others than the patient. This is however little comfort to the patient who is frequently very distressed. Advice to avoid nylon hair brushes, massage and hair styles, which place a physical strain on the hair is all that can be offered. Applications to the scalp of creams containing ovarian hormones (theoretically sound treatment) are valueless. Hair loss due to the breakage of hair without damage to hair follicles occurs frequently from over processing by waving solutions and bleaches. This recovers spontaneously. Loss of hair around the scalp margin is likely to follow the use of curlers in those with fine hair.

Alopecia areata

This is the most common hair disease. It frequently starts in childhood and there may be a family history. Hair is lost over clearcut round areas of the scalp or beard. The bald patches may be faintly pink, but otherwise the scalp appears normal and does not scale. In the stage of active hair fall, broken stumps called exclamation mark hairs are present at the spreading edge of the bald patch but they are absent if the lesion is not extending. Spontaneous recovery takes place in over 60 per cent of first attacks but the prognosis worsens with second and third attacks. Rarely, alopecia areata extends to the whole scalp and even all the hair on the body, and in this instance recovery is unlikely. A bad prognostic sign is superficial pitting and ridging of the finger nails. The cause of alopecia areata is unknown and, though there is some association with emotional stress, this is by no means conclusive. Since the majority of patients with alopecia areata recover spontaneously in 3–6 months, firm reassurance with, if considered

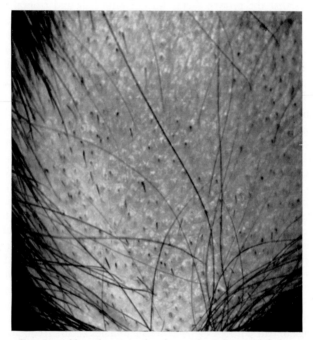

Fig. 82.—Alopecia areata showing exclamation mark hairs.

desirable, a harmless local placebo is all that is required. Injection of corticosteroids into a patch of alopecia areata is usually followed by regrowth of hair and this may be used to encourage both the hair and the patient if recovery is delayed.

The application of betamethasone (Betnovate) scalp application or fluocinolone acetonide, (Synalar Gel) are more acceptable to the patient though less effective than injections. In our opinion, systemic steroids, though immediately effective in alopecia totalis, are not justified and a wig is to be preferred.

Ringworm infection

This is discussed under infections (page 84).

Scarred alopecia

Destruction of hair follicles occurs with any damage to the full thickness of the scalp. Scars from burns, mechanical injury, deep pyogenic infection and radiation can be diagnosed from the history.

A number of rare skin diseases, scleroderma, lichen planus, lupus erythematosis, lupus vulgaris, produce permanent scarred alopecia but they are an insignificant group and need not concern us further.

Hirsuties

Localised overgrowth of hair may occur in or over intradermal naevi and over the spine where it can indicate developmental defects. Excessive hair growth of the face, body and limbs of women is a common and distressing complaint. Some increase of facial hair growth in menopausal women has already been mentioned and hirsuties can occur in metabolic disorders such as porphyria. However, the great majority of women who suffer from overgrowth of facial hair do not suffer from any demonstrable endocrine or other disorder and the trait is often familial and racial. A probable explanation is an inherited metabolic abnormality of vellus hair follicles which give rise to terminal hairs as a response to normal hormone levels. It is important not to miss some source of virilising hormones but if the menstrual history is normal, a hormonal disorder is unlikely. No hormonal treatment can control essential hirsuties and medical treatment is primitive and unsatisfactory. Destruction of hair follicles by electrolysis is effective for small groups of hairs but is impracticable for a well developed beard. Chemical depilatories give a good cosmetic result but often produce skin irritation. Frequent rubbing down of the hairs with fine abrasive paper is acceptable to many women who do not wish to shave. The technique has to be learnt and the patient encouraged in the early stages.

CHAPTER 21

BULLOUS ERUPTIONS

MANY common and relatively harmless conditions are characterised by bullae which form as a result of marked inflammatory oedema in the upper dermis whereas the blisters in some of the less common disorders are due to abnormalities of adhesion between the layers of the skin. We feel it necessary to include some mention of the types of pemphigus, despite their rarity, as, until the coming of corticosteroids, they were invariably fatal and their early recognition and adequate treatment is important.

The following classification, according to age, includes many of the rare conditions which are beyond the scope of this book. The great majority of patients who show bullae will be suffering from diseases in the first column:

	Common	*Uncommon*
Infancy:	Impetigo. (Pemphigus neonatorum)	Congenital porphyria. Epidermolysis bullosa. Ichthyosiform erythrodermia. Bloch Sulzberger syndrome. Urticaria pigmentosa. Congenital syphilis.
Childhood:	Impetigo. Bullous papular urticaria. Erythema multiforme.	Infantile dermatitis herpetiformis. Bullous drug eruptions.
Adult:	Insect bites. Erythema multiforme. Bullous drug eruptions. Bullous eczematous eruptions.	Bullous plant eruptions. Dermatitis herpetiformis. Herpes gestationis. Subcorneal pustular eruption. Pemphigus group. Porphyria. Leukaemic and carcinomatous bullous eruptions. Familial benign pemphigus.
Old age:	Bullous pemphigoid.	Benign mucous membrane pemphigus. Bullae complicating cerebral vascular accidents.

Pemphigus vulgaris

This extremely rare disease mainly affects the middle-aged and has a high incidence in Jews. Flaccid bullae which rapidly become painful erosions occur in the mouth, conjunctiva or vulva some months before the onset of a skin eruption. Thus patients may be referred first to the Ear, Nose and Throat, Eye or Gynaecological departments.

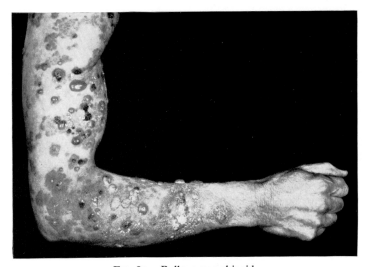

FIG. 83.—Bullous pemphigoid.

Crops of bullae then appear on the skin and speedily rupture to leave raw erosions which show little evidence of healing. The diagnosis can be confirmed by histological examination of an early bulla which will show an intraepidermal split containing disintegrated acantholytic epidermal cells. Further confirmation may be obtained by the demonstration by immunofluorescent techniques of antibodies to epidermis in the patients' serum and bound to the affected area of the epidermis.

Pemphigus foliaceus

A less severe disorder of the same type may present with dry scaly lesions on the face and upper trunk which can be confused with lupus erythematosus or seborrhoeic dermatitis. If this spreads to involve the whole body it can resemble exfoliative dermatitis and the possibility of a blistering eruption be overlooked.

As in pemphigus vulgaris biopsy is necessary for a confirmation of the diagnosis and treatment is on the same lines as for pemphigus vulgaris.

Pemphigoid or parapemphigus

The incidence of this disorder rises with the increase of aged in the population as it affects the age group 65–75 years and over. Unlike pemphigus the skin is affected first, usually by a premonitory itching eruption which can resemble eczema or urticaria. We have often erroneously diagnosed senile eczema only to revise the diagnosis on the appearance of crops of blisters. The blisters which are subepidermal in situation are large, tense and filled with serum or blood and in contrast to those of pemphigus remain intact for several days. The mucous membranes are affected little, if at all, thus it is possible to distinguish pemphigoid from pemphigus on clinical grounds. Histologically the epidermis is intact, the bulla is always subepidermal and immunologically the disorder can be differentiated from pemphigus.

General treatment. Before corticosteroids most cases of pemphigus and pemphigoid eventually died. Today pemphigus can be controlled by systemic corticosteroids in large doses prednisolone 80–180 mg. daily and the improvement maintained on a dose of 15–20 mg. a day but such treatment may have to be continued for years. Immunosuppressive drugs are of value also in those patients who develop side effects from the prolonged steroid treatment. Pemphigoid also responds to corticosteroids and is usually controlled on a lower dose than pemphigus 30–40 mg of prednisolone a day initially and 10–15 mg. a day as maintenance.

Local treatment. Frequent attention to oral hygiene is essential in those patients with erosions of the buccal mucosa. Oral candidiasis is a common complication which may be treated with nystatin suspension. The large blisters of pemphigoid should be drained so that the roof of the blister can settle back into place. Where erosions have occurred non-adherent dressings and the application of an antibiotic cream are indicated. If the general condition of the patient permits, a daily bath containing hexachlorophene aids the soaking off of dressings, lessens the risk of secondary infection and is comforting to the patient.

Dermatitis herpetiformis

Unlike the previous diseases itching, not blister formation, is the striking feature. The itching persists for years and is not alleviated by the usual antipruritic applications.

The eruption consists of urticarial papules and small groups of blisters which are so soon scratched open that it is often impossible to find an intact blister. The diagnosis must be made on the long history, and the sites of the excoriations usually the shoulders, the sacrum, the elbows and the knees. Pigmentation is often present where lesions have persisted for many months.

Often patients have been assumed to have scabies and may have been treated on several occasions with antiparasistic remedies. Biopsy is again helpful as if an intact blister can be found it will be shown to be subepidermal yet have features which distinguish it from pemphigoid. Recent research has shown that two thirds of patients with dermatitis herpetiformis have intestinal lesions similar to that of coeliac disease. Flattening of the jejunal mucosa and a gluten enteropathy can be demonstrated. The relationship between the intestinal dysfunction and the skin disorder is however not a direct one. A gluten free diet is not consistently successful in improving the skin eruption and diphenyl sulphone (Dapsone) 50 mg. twice daily is necessary to control the itching and the eruption. This is so specific a remedy that it can be used as a diagnostic test.

CHAPTER 22

TUMOURS OF THE SKIN

ALMOST every type of cell in the epidermis and dermis is capable of benign or malignant overgrowth but in practice tumours fall into two main groups. Benign hypertrophic malformations which are present at or soon after birth and pre-malignant or malignant changes which occur in old age.

Fine distinction of cell type can only be made by histological examination which should invariably be carried out if the diagnosis is in doubt.

The term naevus has been used to denote birthmarks of all types. This is not wholly satisfactory since pigmented moles arising from melanocytes are also called naevi but attempts to alter custom by introduction of the term hamartoma to indicate tumour like embryonic malformations have so far failed.

Warty naevi

A line of warty overgrowth, the individual components of which are indistinguishable from virus warts, is not uncommon on the face and neck. The warty excrescences are present at birth but the child may not be brought for consulatation until aged 5–10 years. The history dating back to birth and the linear arrangement of the warts serve to distinguish them from tose of virus origin. Sometimes extensive sheets of warty overgrowth may extend down the limbs and occasionally the appearance of these may be delayed until puberty.

Excision is the treatment of choice as recurrence, if incompletely destroyed by diathermy, is common.

It must be realised that epidermal cells can differentiate to form glandular or hair naevi and though not as common as keratinized warty lesions, nodules formed of cells resembling sebaceous or sweat glands and even hair follicles do occur.

Haemangiomata

Vascular birthmarks are the commonest abnormalities of the skin seen in infants. Some slight capillary dilatation which shows as a pink stain over the occipital region and on the forehead and eyelids is present in 25–50 per cent of infants. The majority of facial lesions fade in the first few months of life and the occipital area is hidden by hair, thus no treatment is necessary.

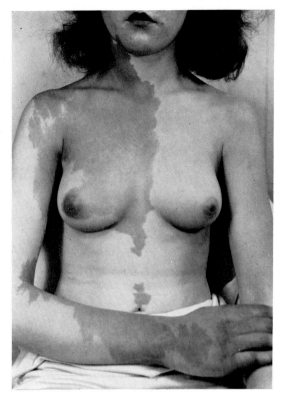

FIG. 84.—Capillary haemangioma (port wine stain).

Capillary haemangiomata

A more serious problem is the true port wine stain or capillary haemangioma which is present in its full extent at birth. This bright purple macular lesion may involve one or both sides of the face, or be distributed over large areas of the limbs.

Although in itself a serious cosmetic defect a port wine stain can also indicate vascular abnormalities within the skull (Sturge Weber syndrome) or arteriovenous communication in a limb which will increase the rate of growth of the bones.

Port wine stains do not disappear spontaneously and later in life nodular vascular excrescences develop. There is no curative treatment but cosmetic creams designed to cover blemishes are now remarkably effective in disguising the disability and should be used when the child becomes aware of the social disadvantage of the disfigurement.

Cavernous haemangiomata

The strawberry mark, so called because it looks like one, has an entirely different natural history from the port wine stain. Absent or present only as a minute red dot at birth it appears when the baby is 2–3 weeks old. Growth may be rapid and alarming until 6 months when it slows down, ceasing finally at a year. By this time, the tumour

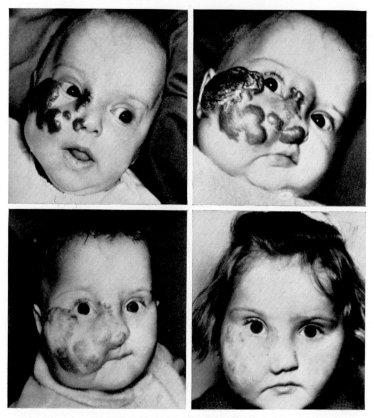

FIG. 85.—Serial photographs of strawberry angioma taken at 3 months, 9 months, 18 months, 4 years. Spontaneous resolution.

is raised and bright red but blanches on pressure. Ulceration occurs in large lesions and in those on the napkin area exposed to friction and moisture. Mothers are always frightened of haemorrhage but this is exceptional and can be controlled by pressure. Spontaneous involution is the rule and this begins at 6–12 months and continues until the age of 8 years.

Ninety per cent of strawberry angiomata disappear entirely without treatment. The remaining 10 per cent leave minimal scars or capillary dilatation and some plastic repair may be required in 1 or 2 per cent. It has been our practice to leave these haemangiomata untreated. Carefully controlled trials have demonstrated that radiotherapy has no higher percentage of success and as it adds an additional hazard it can be withheld. All other methods such as freezing or the injection of sclerosing solutions, diathermy and surgery leave more scar than does natural resolution. The doctor is under great parental pressure to do something but this should be resisted and photographs which show resolution in other cases are a great help in this.

Some angiomata are entirely subcutaneous and appear only as bluish compressible swellings. The natural history of these is not as satisfactory as in the mixed type and if resolution does not occur surgery may be required.

Spider angiomata

One or more vascular spiders characterised by a central papule with radiating capillaries may appear on the face in children aged between 5 and 10 years. They are without significance and can be removed by destruction of the central vessel by diathermy or cautery.

In adults, multiple spider angiomata may develop in pregnancy and liver disease or in the genetic disorder associated with a tendency to bleeding, hereditary haemorrhagic telangiectasia. In a large proportion of people past middle age multiple bright angiomata (Campbell de Morgan's spots) appear on the trunk. They are without any significance and do not require treatment. In the very elderly, acquired angiomata may appear on the red margin of the lip. These, if troublesome and unsightly can be destroyed by diathermy.

Pyogenic granuloma (Granuloma telangiectaticum)

A friable vascular mass of granulation tissue may arise after trivial injury such as a prick with a rose thorn or cut. Common sites are the scalp and the fingers. Distinction between this condition and an angioma may be difficult, since histologically the pyogenic granuloma consists only of new capillaries and fibroblasts. Curettage and cauterisation with electrocautery or silver nitrate is usually successful, though recurrence is possible.

Moles

Pigmented moles are formed from melanocytes, pigment producing cells situated in the epidermis and derived embryologically from the neural crest.

Though occasionally a cause of serious cosmetic disability, the importance of pigmented moles to the physician is the possibility of malignant change in the melanocytes. It should be appreciated that this risk is not great as the average individual has 15 to 20 moles yet the incidence of malignant melanoma is only 1·8 per 100,000 of the population

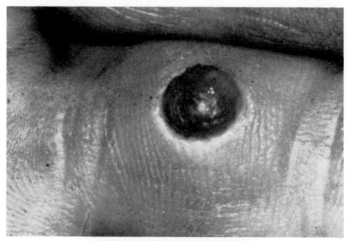

FIG. 86.—Pyogenic granuloma.

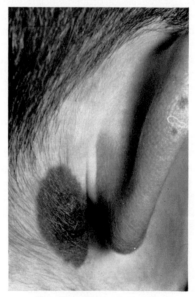

FIG. 87.—Pigmented mole.

per annum. This indicates little more than one mole in a million becoming malignant each year. The incidence is a little higher on exposed parts of the skin and in sunny parts of the world.

Pigmented moles are usually not present at birth but evolve during the years of childhood and even in adult life.

Proliferation of melanocytes starts first in the basal layer of the epidermis at the junction of the epidermis and dermis. At this stage the cells are actively producing melanin and are D.O.P.A. positive. As time goes by, the junction cells drop down into the dermis and become smaller, less active and D.O.P.A. negative. Normally, as moles mature, the melanocytes become entirely intradermal and all junctional activity ceases. The cessation of junctional activity occurs about puberty and, after this time, is an indication of instability of the cells and a forerunner of malignant change.

Malignant melanomas

There is no definite correlation between macroscopic appearance and histological change and it should be remembered that many malignant melanomata do not arise from a pre-existing mole, yet certain generalisations can be made:

(i) Pigmented moles rarely become malignant until after puberty.
(ii) Hairy moles are usually safe and this applies even when they enlarge as many do, particularly in menopausal women. The only exceptions are large hairy moles which cover 20–30 per cent of the body surface.
(iii) The most dangerous moles are the smooth, slightly raised dark brown or slatish coloured lesions less than 2 cm. in diameter.
(iv) As far as site is concerned, pigmented naevi under nails, on the palms, soles, digits and on the genitals are the most potentially malignant ones.

Any change from the normal appearance is an indication for excision and histological examination. Malignancy should be suspected when a mole shows:

(a) Increased size.
(b) Increased depth of pigmentation and its extension into the surrounding skin.
(c) Crust formation or bleeding.
(d) An inflammatory areolar around the mole.

Pigmented lesions which are frequently mistaken for melanomata are seborrhoeic warts which may be very black, pigmented basal-celled epitheliomata, histiocytomata and some angiomata in which it may be difficult to differentiate the deep-blue colour from that of melanin. Folliculitis of the hairs in a simple mole can also give rise to alarm that malignant change has occurred.

Treatment. The legend that to tamper with a mole makes it malignant is not true. Moles can be safely excised and it must be emphasised that it is preferable to do an excision biopsy if malignant change is suspected, since lesser procedures may disseminate malignant cells.

In the treatment of a possible maligant melanoma, wide local excision down to the deep fascia is essential but amputation other than of digits is not usually necessary. It is still a matter of debate whether the regional lymph nodes should be removed at the time of the excision or shortly afterwards, or whether a policy of wait and see is preferable.

Mongolian spot

A bluish pigmentation in the sacral region is seen as a congenital abnormality in the coloured races. The pigment is formed by melanocytes in the dermis. Similar dermal pigmentation is responsible for blue naevi which may occur in the white races on any part of the body. They are much less common than the usual pigmented moles, from which they can be distinguished by their blue colour.

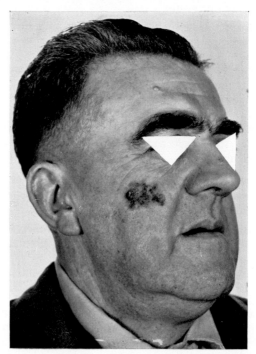

Fig. 88.—Malignant melanoma.

Senile freckle (**Malignant lentigo**)

A dirty, grey black discolouration may occur on the face of the elderly. Slow extension of the impalpable pigment change continues over many years. After 10 to 40 years a malignant melanoma will arise in this condition which, histologically, is a junctional naevus. Here again excision is the treatment of choice but a decision as to whether to submit an elderly patient to extensive plastic surgery can be a difficult one.

Histiocytoma

A not uncommon nodule in the skin of the middle aged, particularly women, is a fibrous lesion which, if examined early in its life, contains many tissue histiocytes, hence the name, and in its later stages becomes a hard fibroma. These benign tumours arise after trivial injury such as insect bites and occur most frequently on the legs. In their early stages they may be quite erythematous, firm dermal nodules, 2–3 mm. in diameter and with a considerable degree of pigmentation which raises the possibility of confusion with a melanoma. The only satisfactory treatment is excision, which is usually needed both for diagnosis and treatment.

Keloid

Another dermal fibrous tumour is a keloid. This occurs mostly after injury to the skin, particularly burns, though in some people they

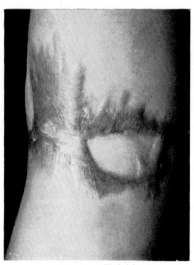

FIG. 89.—Keloid.

arise spontaneously. Dense young fibrous tissue forms in scars which are particularly prone to occur in the coloured races. The diagnosis is simple when the characteristic claw-like formation occurs. Treatment is not easy since excision of a keloid is followed frequently by recurrence. Spontaneous resolution of many of the keloidal thickened scars after burns is to be expected, but resolution may be hastened by injecting them with corticosteroids which we have found reasonably effective whereas X-ray therapy is not.

CHANGES OF AGE

Seborrhoeic wart or Seborrhoeic keratosis

These usually multiple lesions develop on the covered parts of the body after the age of 50. The first abnormality seen is a pale yellow or brown, slightly elevated papule with a soapy feel. Later the lesion becomes more raised with a brownish black warty surface and appears to be stuck on rather than in the skin. Some seborrhoeic warts become so dry and black that, especially on the face, they may be mistaken for melanomas. Crops of seborrhoeic warts often follow an inflammatory

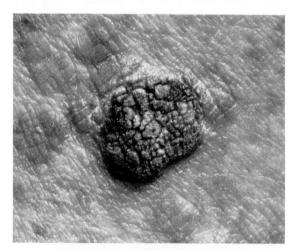

FIG. 90.—Seborrhoeic wart.

lesion of the skin on the trunk such as a widespread dermatitis. Often associated with the warts are pedunculated skin tags which arise on the neck and in the axillae. Seborrhoeic warts are usually symptomless, not pre-malignant and can be left untreated but, if cosmetically desirable, they can be removed by simple curettage under local anaesthesia, followed by the application of cautery or silver nitrate stick or by freezing for 30 seconds with a pencil of CO_2 snow. Skin tags on the neck can be very unsightly but may be readily removed by diathermy or snipped off with scissors.

Senile keratosis

Firm, dry, adherent scales with surrounding erythema and patchy pigmentation appear on skin which has been exposed to sunlight for many years. Such keratoses appear in this country on the face and hands in the 65–75 year old, a little younger in fair skinned who have worked out of doors. In more sunny parts of the world similar keratoses, known then as solar keratoses, arise soon after thirty years of age. Histologically the epidermis shows irregular atrophy and hypertrophy with nuclear abnormalities, a pre-malignant picture. A small number of senile keratoses develop a neoplastic change and squamous celled epithelioma may result. Further exposure to strong sunlight should be prevented and small, non-infiltrated keratoses can be left alone, but if there is any evidence of infiltration the area should be excised. Where irritation is a problem, topical steroid ointments have proved useful.

Leucoplakia

Leucoplakia can be looked on as the mucous membrane equivalent of senile keratoses. It may arise from exposure to sunlight on the lips but is usually a result of chronic irritation in the mouth from jagged teeth and smoking. Syphilis, though a rarity, should be considered if the tongue only is affected. In the mouth, leucoplakia has to be distinguished from lichen planus, a much more common cause of white thickening of the mucosa and epithelial naevi which are usually present early in life. Biopsy may have to be performed to establish the diagnosis. As has already been mentioned, leucoplakia may occur on the vulva where again histological examination may be necessary to confirm the diagnosis. As in keratoses on the skin, leucoplakia is a pre-cancerous change and, once diagnosed, regular observation is vital if it is not possible to remove the diseased area by excision or diathermy.

Basal celled epithelioma (Rodent ulcer)

The slow growing, pearly nodule which is the usual variety of basal celled epitheliomas is the commonest of invasive skin tumours. Occasionally, basal celled epithelioma arise in childhood and early adult life, but the great majority appear after the age of 50. As with senile keratoses, sunlight is partly responsible and the incidence is higher in the fair skinned and low in the coloured races. Seventy-five per cent of basal celled epitheliomas occur on the face and neck but the remainder arise on any part of the body, even the hands and feet.

Basal celled epithelioma should be suspected if the patient complains of a superficial crusted ulcer which has not healed over a period of some months. Often there is a history of trauma, a shaving cut, a burn or a scratch. Because the tumour arises from overgrowth of the basal cells which do not have the ability to form keratin the early nodule is smooth, translucent and without a warty surface. Growth is slow and 1 cm. diameter after 5 years is not unusual.

As the nodule enlarges, a depression forms in the centre and a translucent rolled edge with telangiectases streaming over it becomes visible. This may be made more evident by stretching the skin. Pigmentation

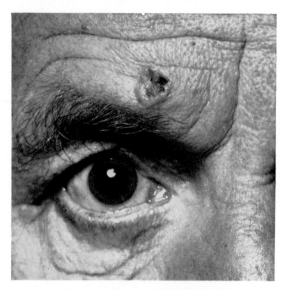

FIG. 91.—Basal celled epithelioma.

may be so marked that a melanoma is suspected. Ulceration occurs late in slow growing tumours which can appear as solid masses, for this reason rodent ulcer is a poor descriptive term. Nevertheless, basal celled tumours are locally invasive and will penetrate deeper tissues including cartilage and bone. Death from sepsis follows penetration of the skull or orbit. Metastases do not arise unless there is a transition of the tumour to a squamous growth, a possible but rare occurrence. The response of the surrounding tissues to the tumour cells is occasionally intense and a firm, fibrous reaction may strangle the tumour cells. The appearance then resembles a scar or patch of scleroderma and the correct diagnosis may not be made because of the misleading history that the lesion was ulcerated but has healed. Basal celled epitheliomas are commonly multiple and may occur in considerable numbers on the trunk where their appearance resembles most closely that of intra epithelial carcinomas (Bowen's disease). They may also be mistaken for the lesions of psoriasis, but close inspection after stretching the skin will reveal the raised pearly margin.

Treatment. The prognosis of basal celled epithelioma, if treated early, is excellent, in the region of 98 per cent clinical cure should be obtained. It is therefore important that a correct diagnosis should be reached as soon as possible. It is essential to carry out a biopsy if a clinical diagnosis cannot be reached. For small basal celled lesions, excision is the treatment of choice, since tissue is obtained for histology and the whole tumour is removed. Larger lesions may be treated successfully by a number of methods and the decision which to use must depend on the availability of the method and the preference of the clinician. External irradiation by X-rays with fractionated techniques is still the most widely used method and is successful even where there is poor blood supply such as over cartilage. In recent years, curettage and cautery has risen in popularity. This method has the advantage of speed and can be done without transporting patients to hospital. Antimitotic drugs such as 5-fluorouracil, podophyllin or colcemid applied to the lesion will alone cause resolution, but their main use is in the very elderly who refuse more active measures. Synkamin, a vitamin K compound, can also be used as an adjunct to curette and cautery or by itself. Where X-rays or other methods have failed, complete removal of the tumour and reconstruction of the tissues by plastic surgery may be necessary.

Keratoacanthoma

This tumour is not as common as basal celled growths but affects the same areas of the body, mainly the central face and the backs of the hands. It arises by the rapid proliferation of squamous epidermal cells, possibly from the hair follicles. Similar tumours have been produced experimentally in animals and birds by application of carcinogens which initiate growth most rapidly in the resting hair follicles. As in other malignant skin tumours, excessive exposure to sunlight increases incidence. The striking feature of keratoacanthomata is that the tumours grow very rapidly and then, after several weeks, involute spontaneously.

The tumour starts as a firm, skin coloured or red papule which grows very speedily attaining a size of 2 cm. diameter in 3 to 6 weeks. As it reaches full size, the centre of the dome-shaped nodule becomes filled with a firm keratin plug and resembles a giant molluscum contagiosum lesion. The sides of the nodule are white or skin coloured with fine telangiectatic blood vessels running over them and in this way resembles a rodent ulcer. The speed of growth of the ketatoacanthomata should help to distinguish them. After several weeks the lesion shrinks. The central keratin plug separates and a crater is revealed which ultimately leaves a depressed scar with a crenelated edge. Keratoacanthomata may be multiple and sometimes appear in large numbers. Both microscopically and macroscopically it may be impossible to distinguish keratoacanthomata from a well differentiated squamous epithelioma and the most helpful diagnostic feature is the extremely rapid growth of the keratoacanthoma.

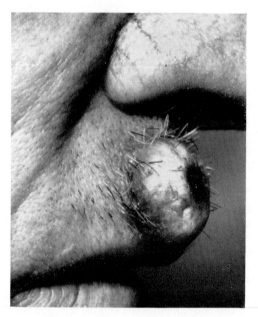

FIG. 92.—Keratoacanthoma of lip.

Treatment. Keratoacanthoma should be treated as natural resolution leaves an ugly scar and histological examination is essential to exclude a squamous epithelioma. A small biopsy comparable to a slice of cake should be taken and the remainder of the lesion can be removed by curettage, the bleeding being controlled by cauterisation. Patients should be observed until the lesion has healed as recurrences do arise.

Squamous epithelioma

True squamous epithelioma usually arises in skin which has become "unstable" as a result of chronic inflammation. Thus it is to be suspected when a heaped up nodule arises in a senile keratosis, a scarred patch of lupus or on the vulva or lip which is the site of leucoplakia.

The tumour arises from the prickle cells of the epidermis and thus can form keratin and in contrast to basal celled tumours is hard and warty. A heaped up, ulcerated cauliflower-like appearance appears at a later stage. Fortunately, most squamous epitheliomas are well differentiated and metastasise late.

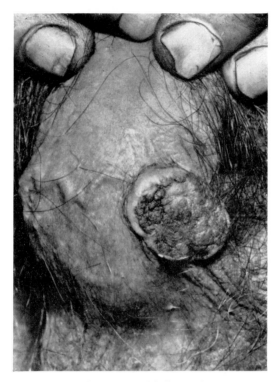

FIG. 93.—Squamous epithelioma of scrotum.

The diagnosis should be confirmed by biopsy and treatment should be arranged in collaboration with surgeon and radiotherapist.

Intra-epidermal carcinoma

A rare, slowly progressive, malignant change confined for many years to the epidermis alone may present in a number of ways depending on the site involved. Bowen's disease or intra-epidermal carcinoma of the skin resembles a patch of chronic eczema or psoriasis. The fact that the lesion has been present 10–25 years and steadily enlarges should arouse suspicion that it is not a simple skin reaction. A true metastasing squamous change takes place when the neoplastic cells burst through the basal layer so a sudden acceleration of the lesion is to be expected. Comparable persistent inflammatory patches can occur on the glans penis (erythroplasia) and vulva. Paget's disease of the nipple is a similar disorder which arises in association with a duct carcinoma of the underlying breast. A unilateral chronic eczema of the nipple and its areola should always be suspect. Final diagnosis of all these conditions will depend on histological examination.

Treatment of Bowen's disease and erythroplasia is by excision, radiotherapy or freezing with carbon dioxide snow: locally applied antimitotic drugs have proved more effective in this condition than in most other neoplasms of the skin. Amputation of the breast is the treatment for Paget's disease of the nipple.

Metastatic carcinoma

Few of the tumour cells which can be demonstrated in the peripheral blood arising from systemic carcinoma give rise to secondary deposits in the skin, but it should be appreciated that nodular growths in the skin may not always be primary tumours of the skin itself but secondary deposits from an internal organ. The correct diagnosis of a solitary nodule is unlikely to be made without histological examination.

CHAPTER 23

GENETIC DISORDERS

MANY references have been made already to the importance of the family history which may indicate an inherited liability to the common disorders of the skin such as psoriasis and atopic eczema. A large number of less common skin conditions are also caused by genetic defects which involve enzyme processes either in the skin or in the metabolism of other systems which then influence the skin. Some of the skin abnormalities are unimportant trivial defects, but others produce severe disability or disfigurement, or indicate systemic metabolic disorders. It is not necessary to acquire a knowledge of all the "rare stamp" syndromes but an awareness of their existence and possible modes of inheritance can be elicited in the history. The inherited pattern of disorders with a simple dominant trait can be discovered easily since affected members will occur in every generation, and approximately 50 per cent of the offspring of an affected individual will show the disease; those not involved will not transmit the complaint. In some instances a smaller proportion than 50 per cent is affected and a generation may be skipped. This is termed incomplete penetrance.

In recessive inheritance affected children are born to apparently normal parents and the possibility of a genetic disorder may be suspected only if two siblings are abnormal. Because recessive disorders are due to intermarriage of individuals both carrying a rare trait, consanguinity increases the risk. Some conditions can be inherited both as a dominant and a recessive trait and as a generalisation the recessive disease has the more severe manifestations. The possibility of a fresh mutation should be considered where no family history of a disorder usually inherited as a dominant can be obtained. Apart from autosomal transmission there is today an increased knowledge of chromosomal aberration, though this has not yet been demonstrated in pure skin disorders. It is important to appreciate that many genetic disorders are not visible at birth but appear in childhood, at puberty, or even in middle age. It is not practicable to list the numerous genetic disorders but mention will be made of several which are either seen frequently or which illustrate some noteworthy feature.

Ichthyosis

The disorders of keratin formation in which there is also reduction of sweat and sebaceous secretion are common genetic malformations

195

of the skin. When inherited as an autosomal dominant the skin change ichthyosis vulgaris is not noticed until after the first three months of life and is often associated with atopic eczema. The extensor surfaces of the limbs are covered with dry scales which resemble fish or lizard skin (hence the name) and characteristically the axillae and elbow flexures are usually unaffected. On the outer aspects of the arm and thighs the dry hyperkeratosis may affect especially the follicles giving the impression of a nutmeg grater. There is usually some improvement in the condition at puberty but it becomes more troublesome again in old age and painful cracks occur over the joints in cold weather. The sex-linked recessive variety which affects males only can be differentiated from ichthyosis vulgaris on clinical grounds as it starts soon after birth, affects all parts of the body and the scales are noticeably large and dark.

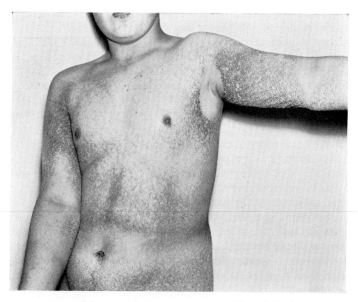

FIG. 94.—Ichthyosis demonstrating the sparing of the flexures.

The autosomal recessive varieties in common with many other skin disorders are more severe than the dominant type and may be lethal to the foetus. When the new-born infant is affected erythema is present in addition to scaling and the child may appear to be enveloped in a coating of collodion or parchment and this condition is called lamellar ichthyosis. The erythema persists until later life and as a result is termed ichthyosiform erythroderma.

Treatment. There is no curative treatment and neither vitamin A nor thyroid extract, which have been advocated on the basis that deficiency of either makes the skin dry, are of value. Hydration of the keratin by bathing followed by an emollient cream such as aqueous ointment or Boots E. 45 are palliative and can be made even more effective by occlusive polythene at night but the condition recurs immediately treatment is stopped. Salt water bathing is sometimes a help and in recent years it has been appreciated that 10% urea in Ung. Emulsificans or a similar proprietary remedy calmurid are more effective than a simple emollient. Retinoic acid, a very unstable compound related to vitamin A does temporarily improve patients with ichthyosiform erythroderma and sex-linked ichthyosis when used in a concentration of 0.1% in soft paraffin.

Palmar and plantar keratosis (Tylosis)

Localised thickening of the skin on the palms and soles is another comparatively common disorder inherited as a dominant. Such thickening may be present soon after birth or it may appear only in adult life; in the mildest examples only if manual work is done. Various patterns of keratosis, diffuse, linear or punctate have been described. The most severely affected patients are considerably disabled and again no curative treatment exists.

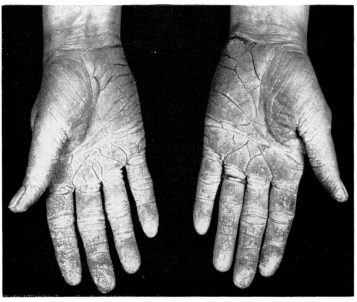

Fig. 95.—Hyperkeratosis of the palms (Tylosis).

Epidermolysis bullosa

This is an uncommon disease characterised by the formation of blisters after friction or minor trauma, due to defective adherence of epidermis and dermis. As in ichthyosis, there are a number of clinical varieties which can be inherited either in dominant or recessive forms. The mildest type consists of blister formation on the feet in hot weather and the onset may be delayed until adult life. Simple epidermolysis bullosa may be noticed soon after birth when blisters form on skin exposed to the trauma of delivery or, more often, blisters occur when the child starts to crawl. Scarring is minimal and the liability to blister formation lessens with age. Blisters in the more severe dystrophic forms are deeper in the dermis and form extensive scars which contain milia (epidermal cysts). Mucous membrane lesions also leave scars which can give rise to strictures of the pharynx and oesophagus. Treatment consists of protection against trauma and the control of pyogenic infection on the ulcerated areas. The control of blister formation by systemic corticosteroids may be necessary in the severe dystrophic varieties as a life saving measure.

The close association between the epidermis and the nervous system is reflected in the number of genetic disorders which affect both. It may well be that the recognition of the skin lesion will aid in the diagnosis of the neurological condition.

Tuberous sclerosis (Epiloia)

This is an association of fibrous tumours in the cerebral cortex which cause epilepsy and mental deficiency and both epidermal and dermal skin tumours. The disease is transmitted as an irregular dominant but

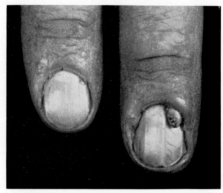

FIG. 96.—Fibrous outgrowth of nail fold, in tuberose sclerosis.

"forme fruste" are common and only part of the syndrome may occur in any one individual. The skin tumours on the face known as adenoma sebaceum appear in childhood, as a cluster around the nose. The colour of the papules vary from faintly pink to red with obvious telangiectases which form a network over and around the papules. Another useful diagnostic aid is the occurrence of fibrous outgrowths from the nail folds and beneath the nails on fingers and toes. Fibrous collagen plaques are frequently present in the lumbar region and these irregular thickenings of the dermis must be sought by palpation. The discovery of any one of these in a patient with epilepsy or mental deficiency should raise the suspicion of tuberous sclerosis.

Neurofibromatosis

Another better known example of a genetic disorder of skin and nervous system is von Recklinghausen's disease. The most frequent signs are multiple pale fawn patches of pigmentation and these may be present alone in several members of a family. At puberty, skin tumours arise from the Schwann cells of the cutaneous nerves. The tumours start as pea sized, soft, faintly pink or bluish elevations. Some continue to grow and become pedunculated, others atrophy, giving rise to curious flaccid sacs. Of much greater significance is the growth of neurofibromata on cranial nerves or in the spinal canal and a possible later sarcomatous change in the tumours.

Many of the inherited defects of the skin are caused by deficiencies of enzymes essential to the normal metabolic process of the body and skin changes may be the cardinal signs which lead to recognition of such a disorder.

Porphyria

The inheritance of a number of inborn errors of porphyrin metabolism is associated with a variety of skin lesions. Erythropoetic protoporphyria in which protoporphyrins are present in excess in the red blood cells, plasma and faeces is inherited as a dominant. Exposure to sunlight is followed by burning and tingling and an urticarial swelling of the hands and face may occur. The signs quickly fade and the diagnosis may have to be suspected from the history. Confirmation of the diagnosis can be made by the demonstration of fluorescence in red cells when they are examined under a lamp emitting 400 nm.

Hepatic porphyria is also an inherited defect which may remain latent until the patient is exposed to hepatotoxic chemicals the commonest being alcohol. The skin lesions consist of blisters, scars and milia on the light-exposed areas very similar to those seen in epidermolysis bullosa. In fact trauma as well as sunlight may produce blistering. Pigmentation and overgrowth of lanugo hair is often present on the face. Porphyrin excretion in the faeces is usually excessive but the presence of porphyrins in the urine is intermittent. The usual test, the finding of red fluorescence under Wood's light therefore may not be positive. Repeated examination of faecal levels of coproporphyrin may be necessary to establish the presence of excessive amounts and to confirm the diagnosis. It is important for patients with porphyria to be warned not to take drugs such as barbiturates, sulphonamides, griseofulvin and the contraceptive pill. Successful amelioration of symptoms can be achieved if the excessive body iron stores can be removed by frequent bleeding or by chelating agents.

Phenylketonuria

Though rare, this condition is worthy of mention since it illustrates well a clear cut enzyme deficiency inherited as a recessive trait and occurring most frequently in cousin marriages. The clinical picture is of an irritable, miserable infant with an eczematous eruption indistinguishable from infantile eczema. Untreated, there is progressive mental deterioration. The metabolic defect is an inability to convert the amino-acid phenylalanine to tyrosine with the effect that a large amount of phenylalanine accumulates in the blood and it is excreted in the urine as phenylpyruvic acid. From the practical point of view all infants should have the urine tested with ferric chloride in the form of Phenistix and this test should be employed especially in babies with infantile eczema. Treatment with a diet low in phenylalanine does offer some hope of success if started sufficiently early.

The hyperlipoproteinaemias

The occurrence of xanthomata, deposits of lipid material in the skin may indicate a disorder of lipoproteins. The most common of these fatty lesions are the soft chamois leather like plaques on the eyelids (xanthelasma) but fortunately less than half the patients with xanthelasma have any evidence of metabolic disorder. The purely cosmetic problem can be solved by the removal of the fatty tissue by excision or diathermy. Far more ominous are the true tumour-like nodules over the bony prominences of the knees, elbows and fingers. Xanthomata also occur in tendon sheaths where they appear as hard nodules, and streaks of yellow material can be observed in the palmar creases and another association is the formation of a premature arcus senilis of the cornea. Though harmless in themselves, the xanthomata indicate either an inherited disorder which may be, associated with an increased risk of ischaemic heart disease or they may arise as a secondary phenomenon in the course of systemic disease such as biliary cirrhosis, the nephrotic syndrome or diabetes.

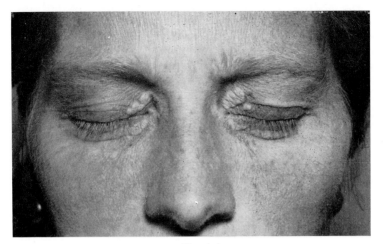

FIG. 97.—Xanthelasma.

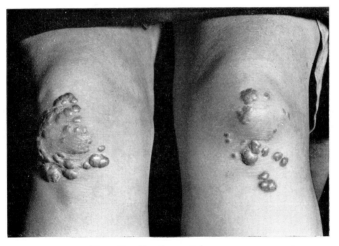

FIG. 98.—Xanthoma tuberosum.

202 GENETIC DISORDERS

The inherited abnormalities of lipoproteins have recently been classified into five different types on the basis of their electrophoretic patterns though they also differ genetically. Prognosis and treatment varies with the correct diagnosis of the disorder, thus full investigation of a patient with xanthomata is essential. It is certainly possible, by the use of diet plus cholestyramine or clofibrate, dependent on the variety of the disorder, to control the hereditary hyperlipoproteinaemia and cause resolution of the xanthomata. Whether early treatment can prevent or arrest the vascular disease remains unknown.

APPENDIX

THE dermatologist is usually confused by the multiplicity of medicaments which are found in even the simplest pharmacopoeia; yet successful treatment of all the common diseases can be achieved by the use of a very small number of topical applications. Dermatologists, like cooks, have their favourite recipes and listed below are a minimum number of our favourite prescriptions and techniques with their main indications and a very brief description of the principles upon which the vehicles work. The methods by which they should be applied have been described elsewhere in the book but explanation to the patient of how medicaments should be used is an essential part of the treatment all too often omitted.

Lotions

Lotions are used to cool inflamed skin and act by evaporation, thus should be reapplied frequently on gauze or linen, never lint.

For acute exudative conditions and general anti-inflammatory use:

Wet dressing of shake lotions:

Lotion terra silica.

White Fuller's earth	4·5
Zinc oxide	4·5
Glycerin	2·5
Water to	100

or calamine lotion B.P.

In endogenous eczema $\frac{1}{4}\%$ of crude coal tar may be added to the lotion as an anti-pruritic but should be mixed with the glycerin alone in the course of preparation. It should not be used in contact dermatitis as the tar may be irritating.

If pyogenic infection is present wet dressings of $\frac{1}{4}$ strength sodium hypochlorite dilute solution B.P.C. (Milton) is clean and effective.

Pastes

These are a suspension of powder in a greasy base, usually soft paraffin.

203

For subacute and chronic dermatitis:

Lassar's paste (Zinc and Salicylic acid paste B.P.)

Salicylic acid	2
Zinc oxide	25
Starch powder	25
Soft paraffin	100

Crude coal tar can be added as an anti-pruritic, 1% or 6% being the most useful strengths.

In the most severe cases:

Coal tar and Zinc Ointment B.P.C.

Strong coal tar solution	10
Zinc oxide	30
Yellow soft paraffin	60

Creams

Creams are of two types, water in oil emulsions which are greasy and less easily soluble in water. Oily cream B.P. is an example of this type useful for dry skins. Oil in water emulsions are easily removable by water and particularly applicable for hairy areas. Aqueous cream B.P. is an example which can be used as an emollient and a vehicle for medicaments. In the use of creams for the dilution of topical steroids care is necessary as the steroid may be unstable or inactive in an unsuitable base. For instance cetomacrogol cream (formula B) B.P.C. is suitable for the dilution of fluocinolone acetonide but cetomacrogol cream (formula A) B.P.C. is correct for betamethasone valerate.

Polythene occlusive dressings

The penetration of corticosteroids in the skin can be increased and the anti-inflammatory effect enhanced by covering the area with an air-tight plastic film dressing. This should not be left on for more than 8 hours at a time and can conveniently be done at night. Such treatment should be reserved for resistant thickened lesions and with an awareness that prolonged use of the method may produce skin atrophy and systemic absorption of the corticosteroid.

Ointments

Non-emulsifying ointments such as paraffin ointment tend to macerate the skin but are useful in certain situations.

Crusts can be easily removed by the application of the following ointment thickly spread on lint strips and left in position for 24 hours.

Lead diachylon plaster | equal parts
Soft paraffin |

Hyperkeratotic skin may also be softened by the use of 10–20% salicylic acid in soft paraffin.

Bisgaard therapy

Used in the treatment of severe venous ulcers of the legs. It is a combination of massage and firm elastic support.

Method

1. Moisten the bare hands with olive oil, raise the patient's leg and rest it on a small table.

2. Massage the sole firmly from toes to heel.

3. Massage the hollows behind the malleoli from the foot upwards.

4. Massage the lower leg and the area round the ulcer to mobilise the ulcer from underlying scar tissue.

5. Give passive and active movements to the ankle joint to improve its mobility.

6. Apply a dressing to the ulcer and bandage this in place with a cotton bandage.

7. Apply a pad of gamgee to completely encircle the lower half of the leg. Bandage this in place with a 6-inch cotton bandage from toes to knee.

8. Apply an elastic web bandage (blue line) firmly from the base of the toes, keeping it evenly bandaged by following blue line and leaving no gaps round the heel. The bandage must be applied from the toes to just below the knee.

The patient removes the elastic bandage when going to bed but leaves the rest of the dressing in place until the process is repeated the following day.

Acne vulgaris:

Zinc sulphide lotion B.N.F.

Sulphurated potash	5
Zinc sulphate	5
Camphor water to	100

To cause peeling in severe cases

Resorcin	3–6
Sulphur	3–6
Zinc paste to	100

Seborrhoeic eczema:

A mild cosmetically acceptable preparation:

Salicylic acid and Sulphur cream B.P.C.

Salicylic acid	2
Sublimed sulphur	2
Aqueous cream	96

For dry scaly scalp due to seborrhoeic eczema or mild psoriasis and those who are coal-tar sensitive:

Cade oil	25
Yellow beeswax	12·5
Soft paraffin	62·5

Psoriasis for routine use:

Coal tar and Salicylic acid B.P.C.

Strong coal-tar solution	10
Salicylic acid	2
Yellow soft paraffin	10
Emulsifying wax	18
Hard paraffin	10
Coconut oil	50

For more resistant patches:

Dithranol in Zinc paste $\frac{1}{4}$%–2%

Scalp lotion for psoriasis:

Liquor picis. carbonis	
Water	equal parts
Spirit meth.	

For very severe scalp psoriasis:

Ung. Pyrogall. Co.

Pyrogallic acid	2·5
Salicylic acid	4
Carbolic acid	2·5
Soft paraffin alb. to 100	

For fungus infections of groins and toe clefts:

Magenta paint B.P.C. (Castellani's paint)

For chronic scaly fungus infections:

Benzoic acid compound B.P.C. (Whitfield's ointment)

Benzoic acid	6
Salicylic acid	3
Emulsifying ointment	91

Baths

Tar baths

Liquor picis carbonis 120 ml. added to 90 litres of water. Used to sensitize the skin to ultraviolet light in the treatment of psoriasis.

Bath oil

Added in the quantity recommended by the manufacturer. Useful to grease the skin in mild ichthyosis and to prevent degreasing of the skin in eczema and senile pruritis.

Emulsifying ointment bath

Place 20–40 g. of emulsifying ointment in a basin and mix it with hot water. Add to the bath water (20 g. for an infant bath). Used to prevent degreasing of the skin in infantile and atopic eczema.

Hexachlorophene bath

30 ml. of a 10% solution of hexachlorophene added to 45 litres of water in a bath. Used to help to disinfect the skin in patients suffering from recurrent boils.

Examination of hair, nails and skin for fungus infection

Pathogenic fungi remain viable in hairs, nail clippings and skin scrapings for long periods which enables specimens to be sent to specialised laboratories even many miles away. Scrapings should be obtained from the spreading edge of lesions either with a scalpel or Volkman's spoon. The material can be conveniently preserved dry between two microscope slides held together by Sellotape.

Skin biopsy

This procedure is carried out under local anaesthesia. A characteristic early lesion should be selected and, if a small blister or nodule, removed entirely. When only part of a large lesion is removed an ellipse of skin which includes a piece of normal skin and the transition to diseased tissue must be taken. A strip of skin cut out with a scalpel is to be preferred to a punch biopsy. It is important to include all layers of the skin down to subcutaneous fat since it is impossible to decide whether a tumour is invading the dermis if only epidermis can be seen. The biopsy specimen should be put in fixative (10% formalin) immediately.

Further reading

CHAMPION, R. H., GILLMAN, T., ROOK, A. J. and SIMS, R. T. (1970). *An Introduction to the Biology of the Skin*. Blackwell, Oxford and Edinburgh.

FISHER, A. A. (1967). *Contact Dermatitis*. Henry Kimpton, London.

JARRETT, A., SPEARMAN, R. I. C. and RILEY, P. A. (1966). *Dermatology, a functional introduction*. English University Press, London.

LEVER, W. F. (1967). *Histopathology of the Skin*. 4th Edition. Pitman Medical, London.

ROOK, A., WILKINSON, D. S. and EBLING, F. J. G. (1968). *Textbook of Dermatology*, Blackwell, Oxford and Edinburgh.

SCHWARTZ, L., TULIPAN, L. and BIRMINGHAM, D. V. (1957). *Occupational Diseases of the Skin*. 3rd Edition. Henry Kimpton, London.

TURK, J. L. (1969). *Immunology in Clinical Medicine*. William Heinemann Medical Books Ltd., London.

WILKINSON, D. S. (1970). *The Nursing and Management of Skin Diseases*. 2nd Edition. Faber & Faber, London.

INDEX

Bold figures indicate pages on which the main references to subjects appear.